"The perfect exercise regimen for our time."
Philadelphia Inquirer Magazine

"Pilates has quietly survived all the various fitness trends."
The Washington Post

"Pilates unquestionably gives results."
Atlanta Journal-Constitution

"By the third session I was a convert."
Amanda Hesser, *The New York Times*

Pilates® Method of
Body Conditioning

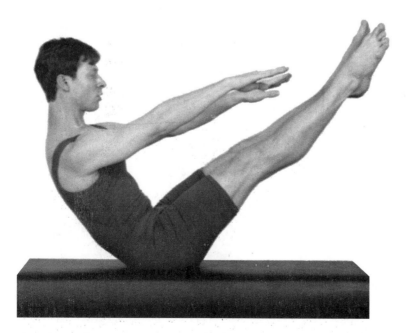

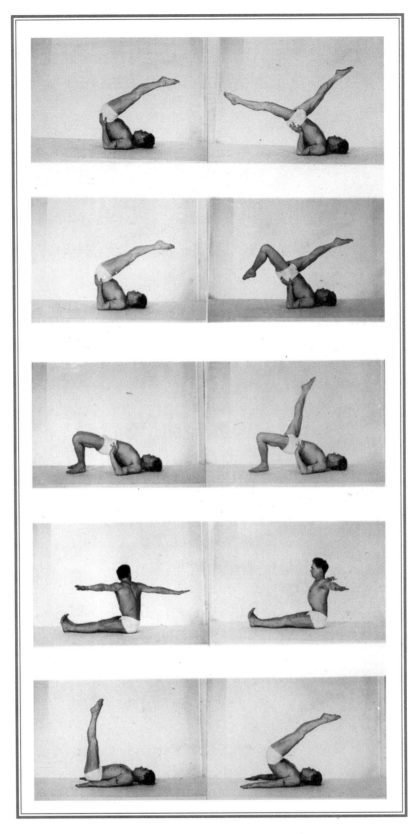

From the Archives of Joseph H. Pilates

Pilates® Method of Body Conditioning

Introduction to the Core Exercises

Sean P. Gallagher

&

Romana Kryzanowska

**Photography by
Steven Speleotis**

BainBridgeBooks

Philadelphia

NOTICE TO READERS

Before following any advice in this book, it is recommended that you consult your doctor if you suffer from any health problems or special conditions or if you are in doubt
about the suitability of any exercise. It is also suggested that you consider consulting
with a certified Pilates instructor before beginning a comprehensive home exercise
program. You may also wish to purchase video tapes that help further explain many of
the exercise programs contained in this book.

Reading this book in no way certifies the readers to instruct others in the use of the
Pilates Method, nor does it allow them to use the Pilates trademarks. Pilates® Method
and Pilates Studios® are registered trademarks of Sean P. Gallagher.

Published May 1999
by
BainBridgeBooks
an imprint of
Trans-Atlantic Publications Inc.
Philadelphia PA
Website: www.transatlanticpub.com

PRINTED IN THE UNITED STATES OF AMERICA
Third Printing, January 2000

ISBN: 1-891696-08-4

Library of Congress Cataloging-in-Publication Data:

Gallagher, Sean (Sean P.), 1958-
    The Pilates method of body conditioning / Sean Gallagher & Romana
Kryzanowska ; photographs by Steven Speleotis.
          p.   cm.
    ISBN   1-891696-08-4 paper
    1. Exercise.   2. Mind and body.   I. Kryzanowska, Romana, 1923-
. II. Speleotis, Steven.   III. Title.
RA781.G34 1999
613.7'1--dc21   98-52214
                                                              CIP

Cover and Book design by: Graphic Decisions, Inc.

Acknowledgements

The authors wish to thank the following people for their assistance in preparing the book. We thank Carol Dodge Baker, who prepared the first training manual for the Pilates Studio®, and Bob Liekens and Sari Mejia Pace for the revised edition of the manual. We especially thank Elyssa Rosenberg for her all-around efforts in coordinating this project and the following people who provided feedback and comments: Ken Bruhns, Fatima Bruhns, Lori Coleman Brown, Lauren Stephen, Penelope Wyer, Juanita Lopez, Dorothee van de Walle, Cynthia Lochard, Debi Crawford and Roxane Murata. We are greatly indebted to our editors at BainBridgeBooks for their valuable assistance in the preparation of the book; namely: Ron Smolin, W. Lane Startin, and Anthony Notaro; and to Peter Glaze and Felix Penzarella from Graphic Decisions Inc. for their captivating design concepts.

Last, but not least, we offer our special thanks to the models in this book — whether instructors or students — who helped to illustrate the Pilates techniques. They are: Zoe Hagler, Leah Chaback, Brett Howard, Stephanie Beatty, Ed Morand, Melissa Fields, and Kathryn Golbeck. And, of course, our thanks to Steven Speleotis for his excellent photography.

Preface

This is the very first book ever published to cover the complete range of exercises designed by Joseph H. Pilates, with all apparatus introduced and demonstrated. We have presented the core exercises for beginners or for those somewhat familiar with the Pilates® Method. All of these exercises can be accomplished at home, however some will require the purchase of Pilates apparatus. The book also provides exercises for pregnant women and senior citizens, as well as suggested routines for those with special problems, such as back pain and poor posture.

If you spend about three hours a week on these exercises, we believe that you will eventually attain superb body conditioning and excellent mental well-being. Quite simply, you will be amazed at how much better you look and feel. You will more easily accomplish your daily tasks and lower the stress and strain in your life.

If you have questions about the Method or wish to pursue it further, please see the directory at the end of the book for the location of Pilates Studios® or certified instructors.

Sean P. Gallagher & Romana Kryzanowska
New York, New York
January 1999

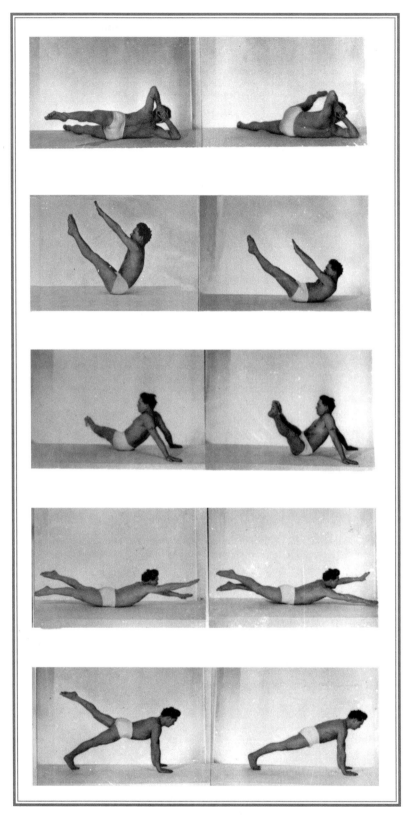

From the Archives of Joseph H. Pilates

Contents

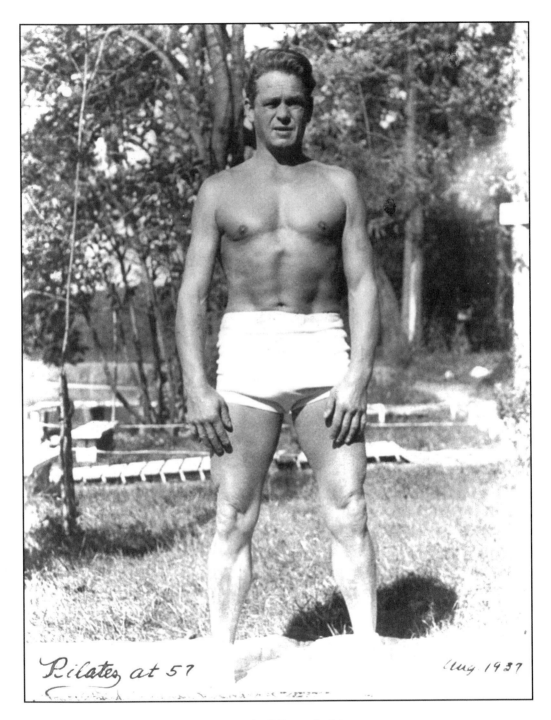

Pilates at 57   *Aug. 1937*

From the Pilates Archives

The Pilates® Method

Joseph Hubertus Pilates
(1880 - 1967)

Joseph H. Pilates (Pi-LAH-teez) was born near Dusseldorf, Germany, in 1880. A sickly child who suffered from asthma, rickets, and rheumatic fever, he dedicated his entire life to becoming physically stronger. In his youth, Pilates studied and became proficient at body building, diving, skiing, and gymnastics. By the time he was 14, he was fit enough to pose for anatomical charts.

In 1912, Pilates moved to England where he earned a living initially as a boxer, circus performer, and a self-defense trainer of English detectives. After World War I broke out two years later, he was designated an "enemy alien" and interned with other Germans at a camp in Lancaster and later on the Isle of Man. Pilates became a nurse in the camp and trained other internees in physical fitness exercises he developed. He was widely credited when none of the inmates succumbed to an influenza epidemic that killed thousands of others in England in 1918.

After the war, Pilates continued his fitness training programs in Hamburg, Germany, where he honed his methods with the city's police force. In 1926, disenchanted with working with the German Army, Pilates emigrated to the United States. On the ship to America, Pilates met his future wife Clara. Upon arrival, the couple founded a studio in New York City which is in operation to this day. Joe and his wife personally supervised their clients at the studio well into the 1960s.

Pilates and his method, which he called "Contrology," soon established a following in the dance community. Such well known dancers as Martha Graham and George Balanchine became his devotees and sent their own students to him for training. Later on, athletes and other performing artists studied under his Method.

Pilates practiced what he preached and lived a long, healthy life, as the picture on the facing page attests. He died in 1967 at the age of 87. Today, his methods and exercises are used worldwide by dance companies, theater groups, students at performing arts schools and universities, professional sports teams, spa clients and fitness enthusiasts at health clubs and gyms. The exercises have become increasingly popular with the general public.

PICTURED AT LEFT: Joseph H. Pilates in 1937 at the age of 57.

Perfect balance of Body and Mind is that quality in civilized man which not only gives him superiority over the savage and animal kingdom, but furnishes him with all the physical and mental powers that are indispensable for attaining the goal of Humankind—Health and Happiness.

Joseph H. Pilates

Introduction to the
PILATES® METHOD

Today people everywhere are becoming more aware of the important part that physical fitness plays in leading a happy and healthy life. And yet true fitness is becoming ever more difficult to attain. Our lifestyles have grown increasingly less active over the last century and thus the condition of our bodies has suffered greatly. We go to great lengths to correct this situation, but these efforts are often met with little or no success. Indeed, sometimes we only succeed in damaging our bodies even more. Why is this so? Because we have lost the sense of natural balance and harmony in our lives.

According to Joseph H. Pilates (pronounced as Pi-LAH-teez), the problem is that people believe happiness can be attained "without that regular disciplined effort required to render our bodies fully mobile, strong and enduring, our bloodstreams pure and our mindstreams continuously refreshed."

The Pilates® Method of Body Conditioning restores this natural balance. What's more, almost anyone can use the system with relative ease: the young, the elderly, the injured, professional athletes, dancers and other performing artists, and anyone else who desires better physical health but just can't

seem to find the time to develop it. The Pilates® Method gives you the body you want safely by leading you to a state of total, balanced fitness.

The popularity of the Pilates® Method among those whose careers depend on keeping fit is a clear indicator of its effectiveness. Some famous celebrities who have enjoyed the benefits of the Method include: Leonardo DiCaprio, Martha Graham, Gregory Peck, Patrick Swayze, Jessica Lange, Glenn Close, Julia Roberts, Sharon Stone, Bebe Neuwirth, Uma Thurman, Terence Stamp, Sigourney Weaver, Joan Collins, Britt Ekland, Bill Murray, Pat Cash, Kristi Yamaguchi, Madonna, Stefanie Powers, NBA player Steve Smith, Tracy Ullman, the Cincinnati Bengals, S.F. 49ers and professional ballet companies in New York City, Philadelphia and Atlanta.

The exercises in this book and those taught at the Pilates Studios® or by certified Pilates instructors are precisely those methods formulated by Joseph H. Pilates.

This system is so easy and safe to use that it is recommended for senior citizens because it tones muscles, improves posture, and helps prevent bone deterioration. It is also excellent for pre- and post-natal women. It can help them learn proper breathing and body concentration and recover body shape and tone after pregnancy.

The exercises stimulate the circulatory system, oxygenating the blood, aiding lymphatic drainage and releasing endorphins which are responsible for the "feel-good" factor. The immune system is given a boost to provide greater resistance to disease and illness.

Who Can Use the Pilates® Method of Body Conditioning?

- Business and professional people
- Athletes
- Physical fitness and training instructors
- Performers and artists
- People who suffer from chronic pain and joint stress
- Senior citizens
- Pregnant women (pre- and post-natal)
- Teenagers
- Anyone wishing to prevent osteoporosis
- Those who suffer from stress and back pain
- Overweight people

What the Pilates® Method is not:

- There is no free play or movements made quickly or jerkily. There is no running or violent movement.

- No heavy weights are involved, and in most cases movements are only repeated a few times each.

- Any straining to the point of exhaustion is considered counter-productive.

- Finally, it is not "physical therapy"...but rather body-conditioning.

The Philosophy Behind the Method

Joseph H. Pilates' method was the product of his lifelong observation of the human body and its natural functioning. He called this system "Contrology," which he defined as "the science and art of coordinated body-mind-spirit development through natural movements under strict control of the will.

"Contrology movements are designed to exercise to its full extension every single bundle in the 800 voluntary muscle-motors each of us has been given to alter ourselves. In fact, the very essence of Contrologic philosophy is that each brain cell is trained to cooperate with others."

The Method combines the best of Western and Eastern traditions, blending the mind and body and viewing them as a unity working in complete harmony with one another. The Eastern approach to exercise is a path to calmness, being centered and whole, with an emphasis on stretching and limberness. The Western approach emphasizes motion, muscle tone and strength. Joseph H. Pilates emphasized these two approaches in his Method.

The Benefits

- Your body becomes firmer and sleeker, with better shape

- You can move more easily and quickly perform many tasks, acquire many desired physical skills, and better prevent injury

- Physical and mental strength and endurance are increased, making it ideal for those working stressful lives or those recovering from an injury

- The mind becomes the body's master, increasing self-confidence and courage

- Most back pain is relieved

- Muscle flexibility and joint mobility are improved

- Strength is added to the body without bulk

- The body's coordination, posture, balance and alignment are corrected

- A good night's sleep assured

- Improved sexual enjoyment

- Fatigue, discomfort and pain are lessened

The Six Basic Principles of the Pilates® Method of Body Conditioning

1. Concentration. You must pay attention to your movements as you are doing them. Always think about each step and you will begin to notice how interrelated every motion in your body is with all of the others. Engage your mind with every movement. Visualize your next step—this will actually help your central nervous system choose the right combination of muscles to perform the exercise! When your mind and body operate as a team, you will achieve an ideal exercise program.

2. Control. It is of fundamental importance to the Pilates® Method that all physical motion be completely controlled by the mind. In other words, motion and activity without control leads to a haphazard and counterproductive exercise regimen. Some exercise programs do not stress the importance of this control. This is why they so often lead to injury.

3. Centering. The human body has a physical center from which all motion proceeds. Joseph H. Pilates called this area the "Powerhouse": the abdomen, the lower back and the buttocks. The Pilates® Method focuses on strengthening this center. The muscles associated with the Powerhouse support the spine, the internal organs, and posture. Virtually all Pilates exercises center on the Powerhouse to stabilize your torso and allow you to stretch and lengthen your body. Centering leads to a trimmer waist and flatter stomach and to a correct posture that can prevent back pain and many other maladies.

4. Flowing Movement. Romana Kryzanowska, the only living disciple of Joseph H. Pilates, often sums up the Pilates® Method as "flowing motion outward from a strong center." The exercises take you through a wide range of motions in a controlled and flowing manner. Do not rush through any step, but rather move smoothly and evenly. You can cause damage by hurried movements. As soon as you feel strain you go on to the next exercise. Avoid stiff or jerky movements.

The Pilates® Method

5. Precision. Precision goes hand in hand with the second principle of "control." Pilates said, "Concentrate on right movements each time you exercise or else you will do them improperly and lose their value."

Coordinate all your movements. After you become familiar with the steps to each exercise and no longer feel awkward, you must command control of your body and seek precise movements every time you exercise.

6. Breathing. Pilates emphasizes the importance of keeping the bloodstream pure. This purity comes as a result of proper breathing during the exercises which oxygenates the blood and eliminates noxious gases. Joseph H. Pilates determined that the best breathing technique for getting out the bad and taking in the good are full forced exhalations followed by a complete inflation of the lungs using a deep inhalation. You will eventually be able to coordinate your breathing patterns with each movement of an exercise. As a general rule, you will breathe in to prepare for a movement and breathe out as you execute it.

Points to consider before beginning any Pilates exercise

Relaxation. Because the Pilates® Method requires control and concentration, many beginners have a tendency to tense up or become rigid while performing the exercises. To avoid this over-controlling tendency, you must relax the muscles but maintain enough tone to hold your exercise positions. You will know when you begin to tense up,

as your muscles will tend to become rigid and shake. Loosen some of this tension to reach a happy medium between rigidity and total collapse.

The Powerhouse. In Pilates, the single most important section of the body is the area between the bottom of your rib cage and the line across your hips, which Joe Pilates called the Powerhouse. Virtually all exercises in the Method work the Powerhouse and lead to a flatter belly and a stronger, evenly developed lower back.

Navel to Spine. This means making the distance between your stomach and back as small as possible. Lie down on your back on a soft rug or mat and breathe normally. Imagine a large weight pressing down on your stomach. Pull your navel towards your spine. Keep breathing without letting your stomach rise at all. Hold your stomach flat while your ribs rise and fall.

Spine to Mat. Lie down on your back, feet together, legs straight. Press your back as flat as you can to the mat (or rug) and remove all the space between the small of your back and the mat. Place your fingers between the small of the back and keep them there, while pressing down as hard as you can. Remove your fingers and bend your knees and move your feet in toward your body. Your back should press more strongly to the mat. Without straining, do this several times until your spine is as flush to the mat as possible.

Avoid Hyperextension. When you extend your arms and legs in Pilates and other exercises, it is common for you to tense up and therefore lock the elbows and knees. This can lead to a reverse bending or hyper-extension, which may lead to injury. Make certain that you stretch your limbs without locking them.

Squeezing the Buttocks. To tighten the flaccid gluteal muscles (the buttocks) there is a very simple exercise to bring back tone and fitness. Whether you are standing, lying down or sitting, imagine a coin between your buttocks. Squeeze your buttocks together so they pinch or squeeze this imagined coin. Continue to squeeze and work the muscles. Repeat this simple exercise often and you will be pleasantly surprised at the results after a few weeks.

Rolling Down the Vertebrae (the bony segments of the spine or backbone). No matter what Pilates exercise you are performing, you must not make jerky or abrupt motions with your back. Joseph H. Pilates constantly emphasized that one should move the torso up and down in a smooth and gradual way, as if you were rolling your spine like a wheel, one vertebra at a time. This will take time to accomplish, but it will strengthen your back and prevent many problems from occurring.

The Box is the posture position in which, while standing upright, you can draw a straight line from shoulder to shoulder and hip to hip.

The Use of Weights

Weights may be used in most Pilates exercises to correct posture and balance, tone loose and flabby muscles and develop other weak areas of the body. Generally, 1 to 3 lbs. are recommended. Never use more than 5 lb. weights.

The Pilates Apparatus

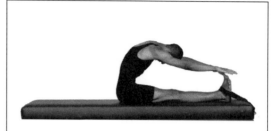

The Mat is one basic foundation of all Pilates exercises and works the Powerhouse including the abdominal muscles ("Abs"). It is the most popular form of the Pilates® Method of Body Conditioning since it is economical and the exercises do not require specialized equipment. The goal of the Mat is to build up a repertoire of exercises that can be performed at home. This program can be done daily. Unlike the other apparatus, the Mat requires you to do all the work yourself and thus is a challenging, but rewarding, program.

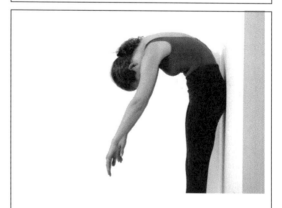

The Wall exercises limber the spine by using the Powerhouse and stretch the hamstrings. They drain tension from the neck and shoulders and strengthen and stretch the thighs.

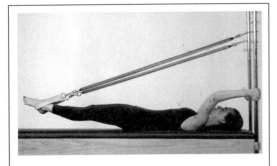

The Springs (or the Cadillac) were created by Joseph H. Pilates and used when working with hospital patients during World War I. They teach you to hold the Powerhouse in place. The Springs are most frequently used for stretching, articulating and stabilizing the spine.

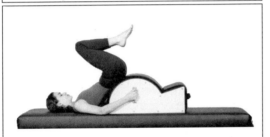

The Barrels help to enhance breathing, develop the arms and legs, work the spine to correct posture and movement, slim down bulky thighs, and massage the lower back.

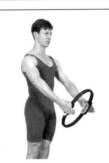

The Magic Circle helps to gain balance and proper posture, strengthen the muscles in the arms and chest, strengthen and reshape the leg muscles and pelvis, and increase control of the Powerhouse.

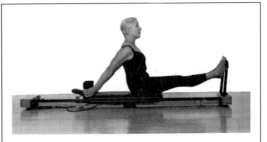

The Pilates® Performer™ is the home version of the Universal Reformer found in all Pilates Studios®. The Performer provides beginner and intermediate level exercises. Advanced work is carried out on the Universal Reformer. Each exercise prepares you for the next activity. The straps, springs, and box provide for a variety of exercises in many different positions. Joseph H. Pilates started all his clients with the Reformer as it is an easier exercise than the Mat. The Mat requires you to fight against gravity and do the all the work yourself. The Performer, using springs, assists you in accomplishing the goals.

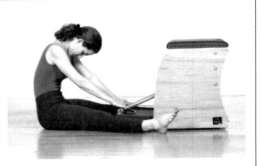

The Chair offers greater balance and control of the body. It offers a whole range of activities including stretching the spine and hamstrings, and strengthening the Powerhouse, legs, feet, calves, Achilles tendon, gluteal muscles, and arms. The Chair is the stepping stone to advanced Pilates work.

FREQUENTLY ASKED QUESTIONS

What is the Pilates® Method?

Pronounced Pi-LAH-teez, this is a low-stress method of physical and mental conditioning practiced for the past 70 years, at first mostly used by athletes and performing artists.

What does the Method accomplish?

To relieve back pain; control weight disorders; relieve stress and stress-related disorders; improve flexibility of the muscles and joints; lengthen and strengthen the body; correct posture by correcting the body's coordination, balance, and alignment; stimulate the circulatory system; oxygenate the blood, thus releasing endorphins; help heal injured tissues; and help prevent osteoporosis (brittle bones).

Who can use the Pilates® Method?

Active people who lead stressful lives; athletes, such as football, baseball and basketball players, skiers, golfers, tennis and racquetball players; dancers, actors, musicians and all performing artists; those with tissue damage; senior citizens; pregnant women; and for all men and women, and boys and girls over 12 years of age. The Method is also very productive for those who lead sedentary lives.

When and why was the Pilates® Method started?

Joseph H. Pilates was a sickly child who suffered from asthma, rickets and rheumatic fever. As a teenager in the 1890s, he began his lifelong quest to improve his health. Eventually, he developed some 500 exercises that helped him and his followers lead a long and healthy life. In 1926, he moved from Germany to New York City and established his own fitness studio, attracting many dancers, athletes, and businessmen.

How is the Method accomplished?

By working out with generally low-stress exercises using different apparatus. This book introduces the core exercises for beginners. Intermediate and advanced exercises are also available — on video, or taught by certified instructors at Pilates Studios® throughout the world.

What is the primary focus of Pilates?

To develop the body and mind uniformly. To concentrate on the Powerhouse, including working the Abs and the upper glutes. To exercise without strain to the heart or other internal organs. To gain power and grace.

If I do not have the Pilates apparatus, what can I substitute if I plan to work out at home or the office?

Many of the core exercises in this book do not require special equipment for home use. If you do not have a workout mat, a rug can be substituted. If you do not wish to purchase the Magic Circle, a ball, 12"-16" in diameter can be substituted. The wall springs can be utilized by installing a set of springs into any door frame. The barrel exercises can be substituted by using small and large pillows. For the Pilates® Performer™ and the Chair, if you wish to work out at home, you will need to purchase this equipment from the Pilates Studio®. These are both reasonably priced. Please see information about all equipment and special videos at the end of this book.

Where can I purchase Pilates apparatus for home use?

All equipment and videos are available from the Pilates Studio® and can be purchased by using the Internet (www.pilates-studio.com) or by calling the Studio at (800) 474-5283, (888) 278-7227 or (212) 875-0189. See information at the end of this book.

Can a person lose weight by doing Pilates?

By using the Pilates® Method, you will tighten all your muscles and lose inches around the stomach, thighs, and buttocks. In conjunction with a proper diet, the Method promotes a lean and graceful appearance.

Is Pilates a cardiovascular workout?

Once you are skilled in the exercises and move through them fluidly, your heart rate will increase and you will sweat, providing you with an aerobic workout.

Can a person do Pilates in conjunction with other exercises?

Yes, there is no prohibition from working out

with other exercise programs depending upon your goals.

Do I develop large muscles with Pilates?

No. Long lean defined muscles are developed.

How many hours a week do I need to spend on Pilates?

For beginners, the recommendation is three days per week. When the exercises are fully learned, this will occupy less than one hour per day.

Do I do Pilates for a certain period of time— weeks?—months?—years?

The ideal response is this: you continue with the Method for as long as you are healthy and have no physical ailments. Many people have worked with the Method their entire adult life.

I have an ongoing back condition. What should I do?

A large number of people use the Method to improve their back problems with excellent results. When you strengthen the Powerhouse, change muscle length, re-balance and relax the body, and correct posture problems, you alleviate many back problems and/or prevent them from occurring. Always consult your doctor before beginning any exercise program to correct back problems.

Can the Method help people with tissue damage?

Yes. Many people with tissue injuries, especially athletes and performing artists, can repair damages to the body using the Pilates® Method.

What age group should use Pilates?

Any age group from 12 years and up.

Can I do Pilates at home or do I need to go to a Pilates Studio®?

You can work out at home (or the office) with many of the exercises. If you purchase some special equipment and videos, you can accomplish most exercises at home.

What costs are involved for home workouts and Studio training?

If your budget prevents you from purchasing certain apparatus, then you can perform many of the exercises with little or no costs. You do not have to purchase a mat (which sells for about $40 with video) as you can use your rug. You do not have to purchase the Magic Circle (which sells for about $30 with video) as you can use a ball. The wall exercises obviously require no cash outlay. Other apparatus, such as Springs & Hooks, Barrels, the Performer™ and the Chair, can be purchased from the Pilates Studio®. The Performer costs about $350 to $400 with video & workout chart. The remaining apparatus becomes available Fall 1999. Please call the Studio for price quotations. If you would like studio training under a certified Pilates instructor, the costs vary between $40-75 per hour for one-on-one training. See the last section of this book for more information.

Do I need to follow a special diet?

There is no special diet required for the program.

What about pregnancy and Pilates?

Pilates is the perfect regimen to prepare your body for pregnancy and to remain flexible and strong while you are carrying. If you are not already training in the Method prior to conception it is *not* recommended that you begin after you become pregnant. However, the Method is ideally suited for post-natal recovery regardless of prior experience. See Pages 180-190.

If I'm a senior citizen, can I do Pilates?

Yes, with your doctor's approval. Joseph H. Pilates used the Method into his 80s, and many elderly people in their 60s and 70s work out several days a week. See Pages 191-192.

Where can I find a Pilates Studio® or instructor?

See the back of this book for a listing of Pilates Studios®, as well as certified teachers.

Does Pilates have a website on the Internet?

Yes. The address is: www.pilates-studio.com.

The e-mail is mrpilates@aol.com.

What is meant by Pilates-based exercise programs?

These use some techniques based upon those developed by Joseph H. Pilates but do not accurately reflect his Method and therefore are not found in this book or in the Pilates Studios®.

How can I learn more about becoming a qualified or certified Pilates instructor?

Information about the teacher certification program can be obtained by sending $5.00 to The Pilates Studio®, 890 Broadway, 6th Floor, New York NY 10003. See website for an overview.

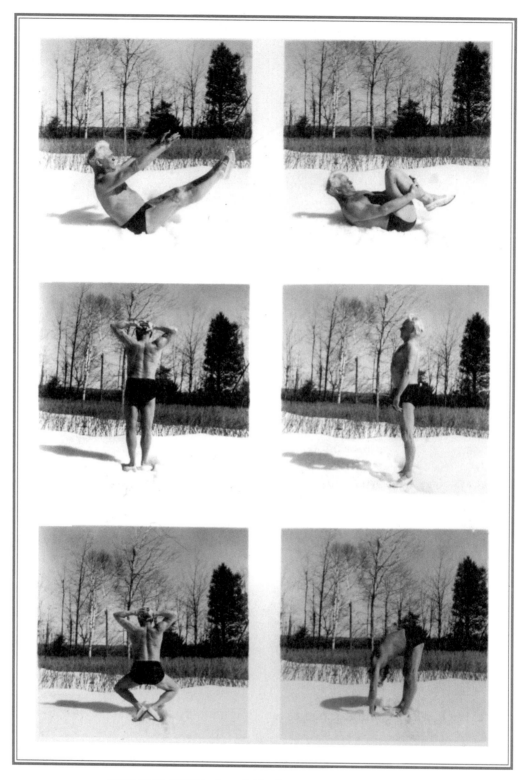

PICTURED ABOVE: Joseph H. Pilates at the age of 77 at his
mountain retreat in Becket, Massachusetts.

From the Pilates Archives

The Pilates® Method and the Benefits of Exercise

by Kara Springer

Making a decision to become physically fit is the first link in a chain of lifestyle decisions. That decision may have been prompted by a doctor's advice, a personal goal, or a convincing article published in one of many magazines or newspapers which constantly present the newest research on the benefits of exercise. Science has assured us that exercise is a necessary part of maintaining a healthy body.

However, the degree of difficulty, duration and the number of times a week required to make a significant change in one's health is difficult to determine. Lately there have been a lot of studies that prove that even the most "non-exercise" exercise, such as cleaning the house, painting a room or walking the dog, can make a significant difference. Even so, it is difficult to determine how much more one would need in order to benefit from quantitative measures of aerobic, resistance, flexibility, and weight handling activities that we think of as "exercise."

One prime consideration that you must be willing to accept when making a decision to become more fit is the fact that exercise must be continued throughout life to sustain any benefits you gain from it. You must make time for exercise and you must enjoy what you are doing so that you are willing to go back time after time. It is not extremely difficult to make time for exercise nor to find a method that is enjoyable to you. However, it is somewhat difficult to allow exercise to become an important enough part of your life that you want, even need, to continue.

Good physical fitness allows us to look, feel and do our best. A good regimen, according to the President's Council on Physical Fitness and Sports, engages the entire human body. It not only works the lungs, heart and motor muscles of the body, but also engages the mind and commands a degree of mental alertness, and emotional stability.

"To neglect one's body for any other advantage in life is the greatest of follies" said philosopher Arthur Schopenhauer. An exercise system that mobilizes a sluggish metabolism into action and more effectively discharges fatigue-produced waste products out of the system is the remedy for the sedentary lives that wreak havoc with our bodies.

The Joseph H. Pilates Method of Contrology

The Pilates® Method was derived from Joseph H. Pilates' technique of Contrology, or the Art of Control. Pilates recognized that the motor functions of the brain controlled the mobility of the body. In his day there was little emphasis on exercises melding the precision of the mind and the anatomical integrity of the muscles. Regarding this as a major oversight, he formulated a regimen that "develops the body uniformly, corrects wrong postures, restores physical vitality, invigorates the mind, and elevates the spirit." He viewed fitness "holistically," taking into consideration the importance of the body working as a healthy unit. He recognized the need for a strong heart carrying oxygen-rich blood to the muscles and forcing accumulated waste out of the system.

Most of the nearly 500 exercises he developed involve a recumbent, or lying flat, position which allows you to exercise without strain to the heart and take advantage of a more natural, relaxed positioning of the internal organs. "True heart control follows correct breathing which simultaneously reduces heart strain, purifies the blood, and develops the lungs," Pilates wrote.

Moreover, the method in its simplest form only demands that you be able to move, even if in the most restricted sense. By committing yourself to execute what you can, exercising the majority of your muscles eventually aids in uniformly developing all of the muscles. "Developing minor muscles naturally helps to strengthen major muscles ... when all of your muscles are properly developed you will perform your work with a minimum of effort and a maximum of pleasure," Pilates said. What is important is doing what you can to reach the optimum of your ability while maintaining complete concentration.

The discipline focuses on the muscles that are considered the linchpin of good posture. The four layers of the abdominal muscles; the rectus abdominis, internal obliques, external obliques and the transversus abdominus, together with the gluteus maximus and lower back muscles, form the support structure for your spine and pelvis, what Pilates called the "Powerhouse." Dr. James L. Oschman, a biologist and lecturer, states that the body battles between the inherited ideal structure and the acquired posture which results from under-use and misuse of the muscles meant to hold the body in balance. The Pilates® Method focuses on the Powerhouse to strengthen muscles which have either been misused or not used at all.

It is truly an all-encompassing technique that can be employed by anyone who wishes to move with more power, grace, and less trauma to his or her body. Pilates builds strong bodies and increases the body's resilience to debilitating effects of age.

How much exercise is needed?
For many years, the prescription for good health had been at least 20 minutes of activity three times a week in order to gain the benefits from exercise. Lately, there have been many experts who disagree with this notion. Recent studies suggest people may not need to engage in this traditional standard of continuous exercise after all.

Joseph H. Pilates originally prescribed exercising regularly four times a week, but he also suggested that beginners limit their sessions to 10 minutes each. "Amazingly enough once you travel on this Contrology 'Road to Health' you will subconsciously lengthen your trips on it from 10 to 20 or more minutes before you even realize it." he said.

The Pilates® Method

What kind of exercise is right for you?

Your fitness goals, present fitness level, age, health, skills, interest and convenient means of exercise are among the factors you should consider when determining your fitness regimen.

The Pilates® Method trains all of the muscles of the body to gain strength in the manner they are designed to perform. Everyone's body has certain weaknesses inherent to that individual. A particularly useful feature of the Pilates® Method is that it will make obvious those places that need more work. In turn your workout will be designed to target imbalances and weaknesses specific to your body.

Most other exercise routines call for an increased intensity, frequency and/or duration of activity over periods of time in order to make progress. The Pilates® Method, however, is more concerned with efficiency. The workout never increases in time but rather increases in the amount you accomplish in that time.

The Benefits of Exercise

By physically and mentally engaging the body in exercise, the body responds by working as a more efficient organism. A pioneer of this idea, Joseph H. Pilates said, "Ideally, our muscles should obey our will. Reasonably, our will should not be dominated by the reflex actions of our muscles ... Contrology begins with mind-will over muscles." This dialogue now has an "engine," a conduit for communication that makes many of the processes of the body work with less trouble, and more effectively for your well-being.

Moreover, people who are physically fit have also been shown to be better adjusted and better able to deal with stress. The brain sends messages via the spinal cord and neural pathways to various parts of the body in order to run, walk and swim. There is a constant dialogue and relationship that the brain must maintain with the body so that we are able to sweat when we become overheated, deliver oxygen to muscle cells, change food into energy and deliver that energy to fuel the cells.

If you or any of your family members have a history of any of the following conditions, they may benefit from regular exercise:

Heart disease and stroke. Physical activity can halve the risk of developing heart disease or suffering a stroke. Exercise helps to reduce the risk of these vascular diseases by lowering blood pressure, raising the level of protective, or "good" HDL cholesterol, reducing the risk of developing blood clots and diabetes and countering weight gain. People who maintain active lifestyles tend to stay healthier.

Cancer. Exercise reduces the risk of developing colon cancer, one of the leading causes of cancer deaths among men and women. In animals, exercise protects against breast cancer. In tracking the deaths of more than 17,000 Harvard alumni, Dr. Ralph Paffenbarger Jr. found that men who exercised at moderate or high levels had 25 to 50 percent fewer cases of colon cancer than the least active men in the study. The main benefit of exercise to the colon is believed to be the increased rate at which body wastes and any cancer-causing substances they may contain pass through the colon in physically active people.

Dr. Rose Firsch at the Harvard School of Public Health found that among nearly 5,400 female college alumnae, those who had been college athletes or trained regularly had about half the risk of later developing breast cancer than the non-athletes. Non-athletes also had higher rates of cancers of the uterus, ovary, cervix, and vagina. Exercise may help battle cancer-causing agents in women because it reduces the lifetime exposure to estrogen, which can stimulate the growth of cells in the breasts and reproductive organs.

Osteoporosis. Exercise at any age can increase bone density and reduce the risk of fractures. There is growing evidence that exercise need not be weight-bearing to foster bone density. Resistance exercise, stationary cycling and water aerobics may help as well. Older people who become active also experience improvements in balance, strength, coordination and flexibility, which all help to prevent the falls that can result in debilitating fractures. Bone is a fluid tissue constantly broken down and renewed. To favor renewal over breakdown, the muscles attached to the bones must be contracted and strengthened. This produces piezoelectricity, a force that results in bone deposition at the stress points. Unless bones are repeatedly subjected to stress, the breakdown process outruns the renewal and bones gradually become porous and weaker. The Pilates® Method can help prevent brittle bones in the elderly.

Diabetes. Older people who are physically active are less likely to develop diabetes than sedentary people.

Weight. The Pilates® Method helps people maintain a normal body weight or, when combined with a moderate reduction of caloric intake, fosters weight loss. Most important, exercise helps people lose fat and gain muscle because muscle tissue burns more calories than fat does. Even among those of normal weight, exercise can counter the age-related loss of lean muscle tissue and the deposition of body fat, especially the heart-damaging accumulation of abdominal fat.

Immunity. Pilates exercise increases the circulation of the immune cells that fight infections and tumors. Physically fit people get fewer colds and other respiratory infections than people who are not fit.

Arthritis. Nearly everyone over 65 shows some arthritic symptoms. Studies suggest regular moderate exercise combined with stretching can reduce arthritic pain and the need for medication. Pilates helps alleviate arthritis and sciatica.

Depression. Exercise has long been known to help people overcome clinical depression. Another benefit of exercise is the experience of positive feelings.

Memory. Even brief periods of mild exercise can result in immediate improvements in memory in older adults. Exercise also fosters clearer thinking and faster reaction time by helping to speed transmission of nerve messages.

Sleep. A study by researchers at Stanford and Emory universities showed that in older adults who were initially sedentary regular exercise, like brisk walking, improved sleep quality and shortened the time it took to fall asleep. After several weeks stamina increased, daily activities took less energy and they slept better at night.

Special Considerations

Generally speaking, if you are under 35 and in good health you don't need a doctor's exam before beginning an exercise program. If you are over 35 and have been inactive for several years, you should consult your physician. "Vigorous exercise involves minimal health risks for persons in good health or those following a doctor's advice. Far greater risks are present by habitual inactivity and obesity," says the President's Council on Physical Fitness and Sports. Even though the Pilates® Method features low-stress activities, if you currently have — or have ever had — any of the following medical conditions, you should consult with a physician prior to beginning any exercise program:

- High blood pressure.

- Heart trouble.

- Family history of stroke or heart attacks.

- Frequent dizzy spells.

- Extreme breathlessness after mild exertion.

- Arthritis or other bone problems.

- Severe muscular, ligament or tendon problems.

- Other known or suspected diseases or medical conditions.

- Back Problems.

Diet. In the past several years the public has been battered by continuous news on what we should eat, in what proportions, in what combinations, and what we should avoid. You name it, and it's been written about. As an individual you will have to experiment to see what works best for you. No one can tell you what is right for your body.

The Mind-Body Connection

One of the most fascinating subjects yet to be fully understood by science is the "mind-body" connection. Many people are convinced of its existence but do not have the faintest idea of how to explain how the chemical processes of our mind are translated into mechanical movements of the body, and even more astounding, translated into feelings, emotions, and memories. Kinesiology, the physics of the body, and kinesthetics, the sixth sense of awareness of the body, may hold the solutions to this phenomena. Not only does the body produce specific chemicals in response to its movements, but the body also manipulates its movements in order to produce specific chemicals.

Meanwhile, those of us lucky enough to be very aware of our bodies, and the ways in which we manipulate them, must continue to use them in ways which produce the effects we desire. This is essentially what The Pilates® Method aims to do.

Bibliography

American Journal of Cardiology, 69: 440, 1992.

Arthur, Stephanie J., "Get Moving." *Women's Health*.

Brody, Jane, et al. *The New York Times Book of Health*. New York: Random House. 1997.

D'Adamo, Dr. Peter J., *Eat Right 4 Your Type*. New York: J.P. Putnam & Sons. 1996.

Diabetes Care, 6: 268, 1983.

Diabetes Care, 17: 1469, 1994.

Gittleman, Ann Louise, M.S., C.N.S., "Healthy Talk: Your Food Health and Nutrition Connection." Premier Issue. 1996.

Kansas State University News. "Heath Benefits from Exercise Programs." News Services. 7, November. 1996.

Journal of Cardiac Rehabilitation, 3:183, 1983.

President's Council on Physical Fitness and Sports. "Guidelines for Personal Exercise." Programs Fitness Fundamentals posted by Hopkins Technology. 1995.

Journal of Cardiac Rehabilitation, 3: 839, 1983.

Journal of the National Cancer Institute, 86: 1419, 1994; Cancer, 1995.

Pilates, Joseph H. *Return to Life.*

Preventive Medicine, 17: 432, 1988;

Nutrition, 7: 137, 1991;

Eades, Michael R., M.D. and Mary Dan Eades M.D. *Protein Power*. New York: Bantam Books. 1996.

Rhodes, Maura. *Women's Sport and Fitness*. January/February 1996. p.46.

www.adamo.com

www.ornish.com

www.pritikin.com

Yakel, Natalie. Health ResponseAbility Systems©, 1995.

Kara Springer *graduated from Southern Methodist University in 1994 with a B.F.A. in Dance Performance. In 1998 she was awarded a scholarship at the Alvin Ailey American Dance Center. She has taught in Dallas, Texas; Vienna, Austria; and currently teaches in New York City. She began her pre-med program at Columbia University in the spring of 1999. After a skiing accident in 1992 she discovered the Pilates® Method and has been an advocate ever since.*

CONSULTING A CERTIFIED PILATES INSTRUCTOR

Although this book provides instructions for home use of the apparatus created by Joseph H. Pilates, in many cases there is no substitute for meeting with a certified instructor to help you adjust to your home-based program. Even one or two sessions with a trained instructor will assist you to gain confidence, find and correct your weak points, achieve symmetry, and develop the mind-body relationship so essential in the Pilates® Method of body conditioning. Pregnant women, senior citizens and those with physical ailments should seek the assistance of a certified instructor in developing a program to suit their needs.

If you would like to work with a personal trainer, there are certified instructors located throughout the United States, Canada, and a growing number of countries around the world. Please consult the back of this book for more information.

The Pilates Studio® also offers several training videos for beginners, intermediate and advanced students. Information about these can be found at the conclusion of this book.

Summary of Core Exercises

THE MAT

1. The Hundred
2. The Roll-Up
3. Leg Circles
4. Single Leg Stretch
5. Double Leg Stretch
6. Single Straight Leg Stretch
7. Double Straight Leg Stretch
8. Criss Cross
9. Spine Stretch Forward
10. Open Leg Rocker
11. The Saw
12. The Neck Roll
13. Single Leg Kicks
14. Neck Pull
15. Side Kicks
16. Side Kicks: Up and Down
17. Side Kicks: Small Circles
18. Teaser 1
19. Teaser 2

THE WALL

20. The Roll Down
21. Sitting on the Chair

WALL SPRINGS (THE CADILLAC)

22. Rolling Back
23. Leg Circles
24. Walking
25. Beats
26. Rond de Jambe
27. Chest Expansion
28. Bicycle
29. Boxing
30. Shaving the Head
31. The Hug
32. Squat

THE MAGIC CIRCLE

33. Standing / Arms
34. Push Down

SMALL & LARGE BARRELS

35. Arm Extension
36. Arm Circles
37. Spine Corrector: Arm Circles
38. Circles
39. Walking
40. Bicycle
41. Scissors
42. Beats
43. Rolling In and Out

PILATES® PERFORMER™

44a. Footwork 1
44b. Footwork 2
45. The Hundred
46. Coordination
47. Long Stretch
48. Down Stretch
49. Up Stretch
50. Elephant
51. Stomach Massage: Round
52. Stomach Massage: Hands Back
53. Stomach Massage: Reach-Up
54. Stomach Massage: Twist
55. Knee Stretch: Round
56. Knee Stretch: Arched
57. Knee Stretch: Knees Off
58. Running
59. Long Box: Pulling Straps
60. Long Box: Pulling Straps—T

THE CHAIR

61. Push Down
62. Pull Up
63. Arches
64. Tendon Stretch
65. The Table
66. Spine Stretch

PREGNANCY

P-1. Modified Roll-Up
P-2. Leg Circles
P-3. Single Leg Stretch
P-4. Double Leg Stretch
P-5. Spine Stretch
P-6. Spine Twist
P-7. Side Kick
P-8. Sitting and Squeezing
P-9. Rolling Down with Squeezing

**The Pilates® Method of Body Conditioning
(Pilates is pronounced: Pi-LAH-teez)**

Articulate

In exercise jargon, this means to differentiate the spinal column one vertebra at a time.

Barrels (Spine Corrector)

The large and small Barrels used in the Pilates® Method enhance breathing, develop both the arms and legs, and work the spine to help correct posture and movement. The barrels can be substituted by using firm pillows, both small and large.

"C" Curve

The torso forms a "C" shape with concavity in front of the body.

Cadillac

Developed by Joseph H. Pilates for hospital patients, springs are used to provide resistance exercises, mainly to stretch and articulate and stabilize the spine. For home use, springs and hooks can be purchased to simulate the Cadillac by using any door frame.

Centering

The main focus of the Pilates® Method, all work starts from the center, or Powerhouse.

Chair

This apparatus helps you to find and strengthen your Powerhouse. It helps to develop the knees and restore your sense of proper balance.

Contrology

This is the name given by Joseph H. Pilates to his series of exercises developed in the early to mid-1900s. It emphasizes the mind's control over the body.

Hundred

This is found in several exercises, the first of which is the Mat, and is used for warming up and working the Powerhouse and increasing circulation. See Exercises 1 and 45

Magic Circle

This is a simple and inexpensive isometric device to firm the muscles of the upper arms, neck, and inner thighs (especially for expectant mothers). This piece of equipment can be substituted by a ball of 12-16" in diameter.

Mat

The most popular Pilates® apparatus, since it is economical and can be used at home, on the job, or during vacations. It a major foundation of the Method, as all exercises are done with natural movements. The exercises work the Powerhouse, including the "Abs," and lay the groundwork for all other exercise equipment. The Mat should be sturdy enough to provide strong support for your back. You may also work on a thick rug with a towel or blanket under you.

Mind-Body Conditioning

The Pilates® Method stresses the blend of Western and Eastern approaches to well-being. The Western approach is dynamic, with the emphasis on motion, muscle tone and strength. The Eastern approach is static, with the emphasis on rest, contemplation, stretching, and limberness. In both methods, the mind can exert great control over the body, while physical exercise can improve many aspects of mental fatigue. Essentially, the Pilates® Method allows the mind and body to help one another.

Navel to the Spine

The mental image and the physical activity of pulling your belly button into your spine, thus engaging the Powerhouse.

Osteoporosis

The development of brittle bones. Common among older people, this condition can be greatly alleviated by the Pilates® Method.

Pilates® Method

Pronounced Pi-LAH-teez, this method was developed by Joseph H. Pilates more than 70 years ago. Some 500 exercises were created to bring the mind and the body together into flowing movements without stress to provide a most effective conditioning program.

Pilates® Performer™

This apparatus is the home version of the Universal Reformer. It provides a wide range of exercises, from simple to intermediate, in order to develop the Powerhouse. It contains straps, springs, and a box for activities devoted to improving most muscles and joints. When you master the Performer you exercise in constant, fluid movement with the minimum of movement.

Powerhouse

(Also called "the girdle of strength.")

The area between the bottom of your rib cage and the line across your hips—for many the most neglected area of the body. Working the Powerhouse, as virtually all Pilates exercises do, flattens the stomach, firms the buttocks, and corrects a weak and painful lower back. The Pilates® Method focuses on specific muscle groups in this center of the body, namely: the rectus abdominis, the internal obliques, lower back muscles, the transversus abdominis and the gluteus maximus—all of which form the support structure for the spine and pelvis areas.

Pilates Stance

Standing tall and lifted with your feet, heels together, in a "V" position. The angle of the opening of the feet varies according to your comfort. "Zip" your legs together. Maintain a "Box" posture (see Page 14).

Roll Down

In exercises where you are asked to "roll down," you must work one vertebra at a time. (See articulate.)

Vertebra

Any one of the bony segments of the spine or backbone.

PLEASE READ THE FOLLOWING BEFORE BEGINNING THE EXERCISE ROUTINES

Caution to all readers:

Common sense dictates that if you have any physical ailments you must consult with your physician before attempting any new exercise program. We also advise consulting a certified Pilates instructor who will assess your problem areas and create a program which targets your special needs. Discontinue any exercise that causes any discomfort or pain.

Caution to senior citizens:

While the Pilates® Method is used successfully by many people in their 60s, 70s and 80s, it is absolutely essential that you speak with your family physician before beginning any new exercise program. In this book there are specific exercise routines to follow for senior citizens. Please read that chapter to find the exercises best suited for you. See Pages 191-192.

Caution to pregnant women:

It is strongly advised to begin Pilates before conception. If you have not done Pilates before, but are pregnant, do not begin any exercises. It is absolutely essential to speak with your physician before starting any new exercise program during pregnancy. Pilates is excellent for post-natal recovery, even if you have never done Pilates before. See Pages 180-190 for detailed information about pregnancy and Pilates, as well as nine recommended exercises.

GETTING STARTED

A detailed, week-by-week regimen of recommended routines is available beginning on Page 194.

1. Warm up. Exercise #1 is the warm-up for all exercises.

2. Never exercise immediately after eating.

3. Do not exercise when you are sick.

4. Do not exercise when you are seriously fatigued.

5. Exercises can be done in the morning, afternoon, or evening.

6. You can break the schedule so that you can do different routines at different times during the day.

7. You can exercise at work if you have a thick rug or exercise mat to protect your back. You can exercise with the Magic Circle at work anytime. Obviously, wall exercises can be performed anywhere. If it is possible, you can install springs in a door frame at work, and perform springs routines.

8. You should not try to perform every exercise in this book in the beginning stages of your regimen. Try only a few exercises for each piece of apparatus and practice daily. Take a week or two until you are comfortable with them, and then you may add additional exercises, but only a few at a time. Eventually, you should perform most of the exercises about three days a week. See Page 194.

9. If in the beginning you feel strain from any particular exercise, cut down on the repetitions until you are comfortable with them and experience no strain.

10. Always work up to the number of repetitions of an exercise. Do not start out by trying to do too much.

11. This book contains suggested exercises for particular problems you may have, such as back pain or posture faults. Read Page 193 to plan a routine to help you improve.

Part 1
The Mat

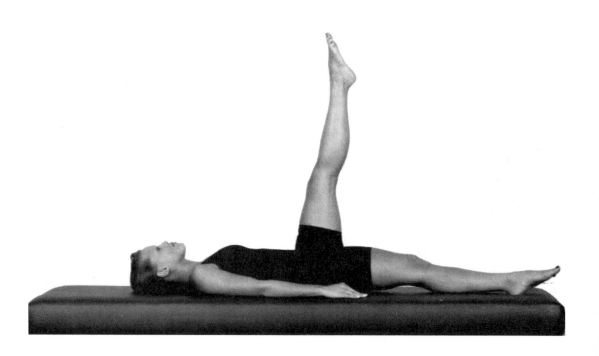

The Pilates® Method

The Mat is the most popular form of the Pilates® Method since it is economical and can be used at home, on the job, or during vacations. It is a strong foundation of the Method, as all exercises are done with natural movements. The exercises work the Powerhouse including the "Abs" and lay the groundwork for other exercise apparatus. The mat should be sturdy enough to provide strong support for your back.

Objectives:

Stimulate the lungs and heart

Articulate the spine

Stretch the legs

Massage spinal column and
surrounding muscles

Work the Powerhouse including
the "Abs"

Strengthen and lengthen the legs

Stretch the hamstrings

Gain flexibility

Rid the body of "love handles"

Improve balance and posture

Release tension from the neck
and shoulders

Work the biceps and triceps

Stretch inner and outer thighs

Develop proper breathing techniques

SUBSTITUTION: Instead of the mat you may also work on a rug with a towel or blanket underneath you

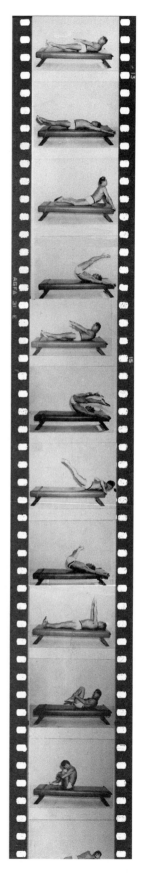

Exercise 1
The Hundred (Warm Up)

A breathing exercise to stimulate the lungs and heart and get your blood circulating from head to toe

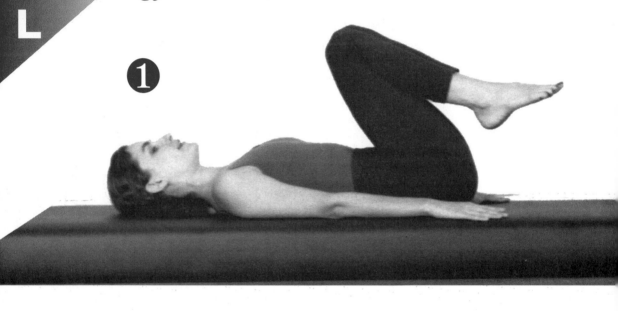

1. Lie on your back with arms stretched alongside your body, palms facing down. Bend your knees into your chest.

2. Lift both legs up to a 90 degree angle off the mat. Bring your chin to your chest. "Draw" the weight of your head into the center of your body. Do not lift the upper body higher than to the base of your shoulder blades on the Mat. Raise both arms about 6 to 8 inches above your thighs.

3. Lower your legs to a 45 degree angle. Inhaling slowly through the nose, pump your arms up and down for five counts. Keep your arms straight and pump from the shoulders only.

4. Exhaling slowly through the nose, continue to pump for five counts. Inhale for five counts, exhale for five counts. Repeat the pattern until a maximum of 100 movements is reached. Relax completely.

The Pilates® Method

"The Pilates® Method restores the sense of natural balance and harmony in our lives."

Sean P. Gallagher

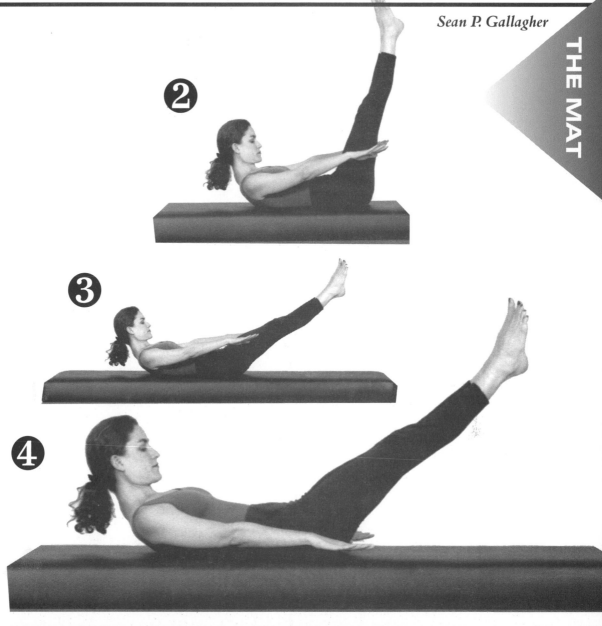

Focus Points

Begin with only 20 movements. Gradually increase until the maximum of 100 is reached. At the first sign of neck tension, place your head on the mat and continue breathing.

Pumping your arms rapidly gets your blood pumping and your breath circulating. Squeeze your buttocks throughout the exercise.

Make sure your back remains completely on the mat. If you cannot maintain a flat back with legs at a 45 degree angle, then raise your legs to a level you can control.

Your waist should be planted firmly on the mat.

Exercise 2
The Roll-Up ❶

Articulate your spine through your Powerhouse

❷

1. Lie flat on your back. Extend your arms shoulder width over your head, palms facing up. Make sure your legs are straight and together. Suck in your stomach as far as possible. Press your navel to your spine.

❸

2. Inhaling slowly, raise your arms toward the ceiling. Keep your stomach muscles tight.

3. Arms outstretched in front of you, exhale slowly and roll forward to a sitting position.

4. As you finish exhaling, continue to roll forward until your upper body is directly over your legs. Try to touch your toes.

The Pilates® Method

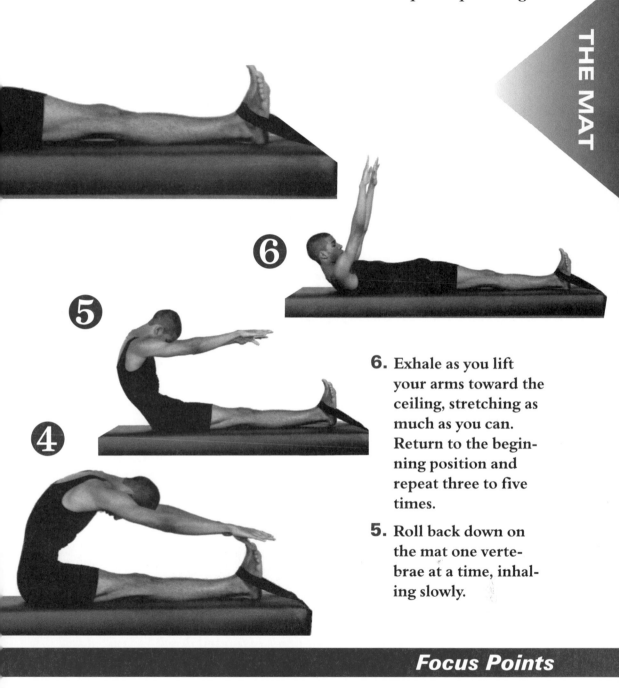

6. Exhale as you lift your arms toward the ceiling, stretching as much as you can. Return to the beginning position and repeat three to five times.

5. Roll back down on the mat one vertebrae at a time, inhaling slowly.

Focus Points

Anchor your feet under a piece of furniture or have your partner hold your feet down.

If you cannot roll up properly, secure your feet under a strap. If you cannot "peel" your back up off the mat smoothly, bend your knees slightly.

Squeeze your buttocks throughout this exercise.

Grasping a lightweight bar, a partner or trainer can assist you by gently pulling you to the forward and back positions.

Exercise 3
Leg Circles

Stretch your legs
while maintaining perfect posture

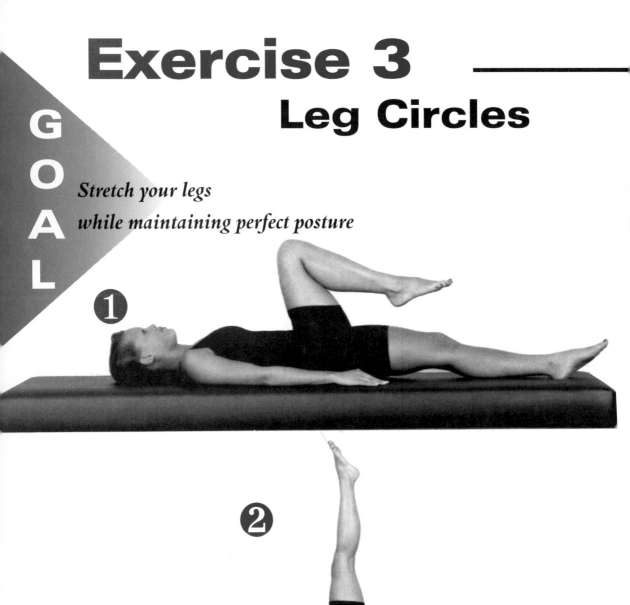

1. Lie flat on your back with your arms extended down at your sides, palms down. Bring in your stomach muscles . Bring your right knee to your chest.

2. Bring your right leg to an upright position at a 90 degree angle to the mat. Reach for the center of your body. If your leg muscles are tight, it is okay to bend the knees.

The Pilates® Method

> *"By the third session I was a convert. I was getting the aerobic workout I wanted while regaining the flexibility I had lost."*
>
> *Amanda Hesser,* New York Times

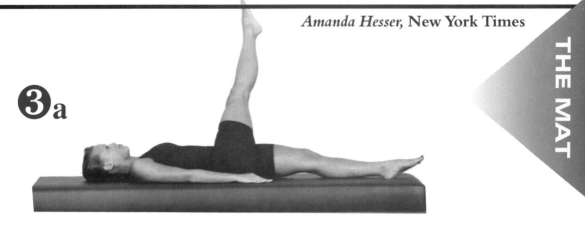

3a

3b

3c

3a. Keeping both hips anchored to the mat, make a circle with your leg crossing over the body first, **3b.** then down round the other foot and **3c.** back to the starting position. Repeat for 5 circles. After 5 circles in one direction, reverse the direction. Then bend the leg and "hug" it towards you, stretching. Repeat with the left leg.

Focus Points

Crossing over the body and reaching up for the center are the most important parts of the exercise. The accent of the circles is on the "up."

Keep the circles small and controlled, in other words, "within the joint." Do not move the lower back.

Make sure your body stays anchored to the mat throughout the exercise. Anchor your a foot under a piece of furniture or have your partner hold your foot down.

Exercise 4
Single Leg Stretch

To stretch and lengthen your legs, open your lower back and work on your Powerhouse

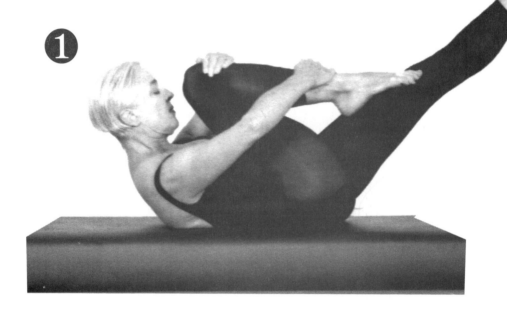

1. Pull your right leg toward you and bend it as far as possible towards your chest, inhaling slowly. Lift your chin towards your chest. Place your left hand on your right knee and your right hand on your right ankle. This hand position is used to keep the ankle, knee and hip aligned.

"Anybody can do it. You can be young and athletic or old and crippled. It doesn't really matter."

Dorothee van de Walle, Seattle-area Pilates trainer

THE MAT

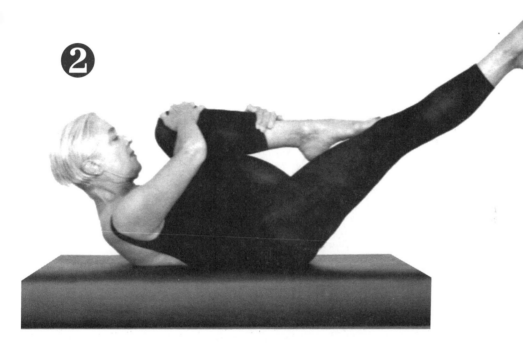

2. Exhaling slowly, change legs and repeat with the left leg. Be sure to extend the right leg out. Repeat between 5 and 10 repetitions.

Focus Points

Point your chin toward your chest. Keep your elbows off the mat and to the sides.

Maintain a flat back. Keep your stomach muscles in.

For people with a bad knee, place your hands on your thigh and underneath your knee for added support.

Exercise 5 —
Double Leg Stretch

To strengthen and lengthen your legs
To strengthen the Powerhouse

1

1. Lie flat with both legs bent into your chest. Pull your lower legs in with your hands and lift your head.

2. Inhaling slowly and keeping your chin in your chest, simultaneously reach overhead and extend your legs out. Keep your heels about 30 to 60 degrees off the mat. Be sure to keep your stomach muscles in.

3. Exhaling slowly, circle your arms around.

4. draw both legs upward into your chest again. Grab your ankles and hug your legs firmly to your chest while deepening the exhalation. Repeat 5 to 10 times.

The Pilates® Method

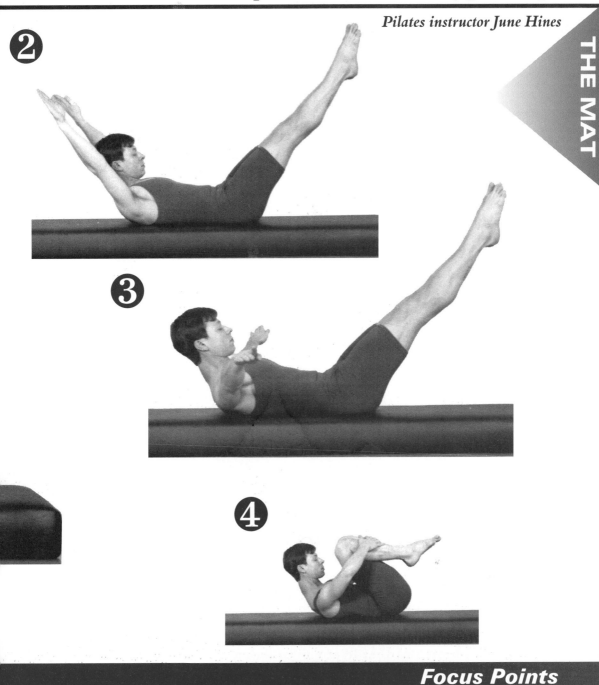

"If you can strengthen your abs and your back, you can control the rest of your body."

Pilates instructor June Hines

THE MAT

Focus Points

Exercise caution if you have lower back pain.

For the advanced version of this exercise progress to lowering arms and legs to 2 inches from the mat.

The stomach muscles are held in to insure a flat back. Extend your legs only as low as you can maintain a flat back.

Pay close attention to inhaling and exhaling at the appropriate times.

41

Exercise 6
Single Straight Leg Stretch

GOAL

A Powerhouse exercise designed to stretch and strengthen your legs

①

1. Lie flat on your back and bring your stomach muscles in. Lift your shoulders off the mat and bring your chin to your chest.

2. Lift one leg into the air and take hold of one ankle with both hands. Point your other leg straight out and about 2 to 12 inches off the mat. Keep both legs in the center of your body. Lifting your elbows to the side, pull the "up leg" with a double pulse towards you.

3. Scissor-like, switch the legs. Keep them straight throughout. Repeat 5 to 10 times.

> *"Pilates is massage and counter-massage to touch all the pressure points on your body."*
>
> *Romana Kryzanowska*

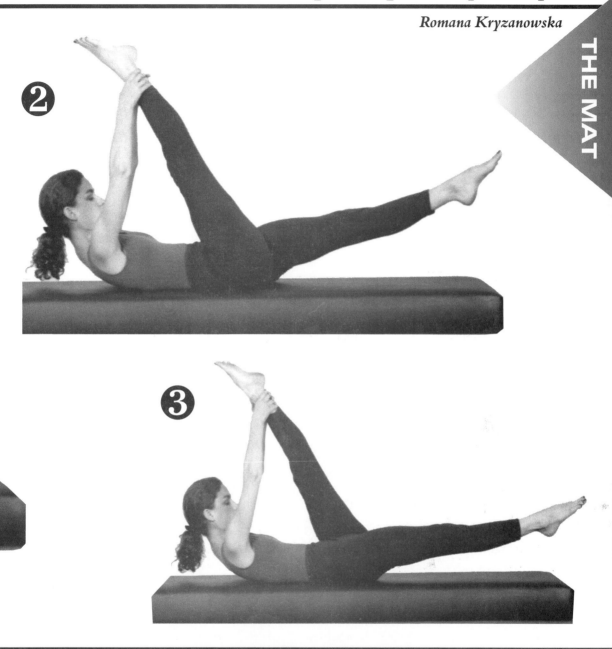

Focus Points

If your leg muscles are stiff pull back only as far as you are able while still maintaining a straight leg. As you gain flexibility you will be able to pull back farther.

Keep the rhythm dynamic as the leg pulses twice towards the forehead and during the leg change.

Make sure you hold your ankle, keeping the knees straight and the elbows out for maximum stretch.

Keep your back flat on the mat at all times.

Exercise 7
Double Straight Leg Stretch

A more challenging leg and Powerhouse exercise for strength and flexibility

1a

1a,b. Lie flat on your back and pull your knees into your chest. Extend both legs straight up into the air. Lift your shoulders off the mat with your chin on your chest. Place both hands behind your head with the elbows open.

1b

"Pilates has made me more in tune with my muscles and how my body functions."

Actor Gavin Lewis

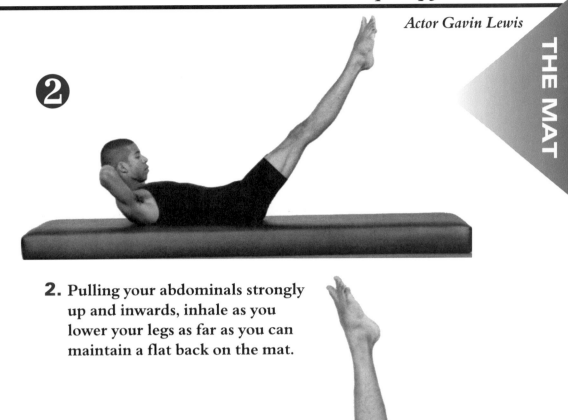

2. Pulling your abdominals strongly up and inwards, inhale as you lower your legs as far as you can maintain a flat back on the mat.

3. Exhale and bring the legs towards a 90 degree angle. Return to starting position. Repeat 5-10 times.

Focus Points

CAUTION: Do not attempt this exercise if you have lower back pain.

Make sure your chin is pressed into your chest and your shoulders are off the mat. Make the Powerhouse work to stabilize the pelvis as the legs lower and lift.

Move legs toward floor to 45 degree angle and then raise them quickly while pulling the stomach into the back.

Exercise 8
Criss Cross

To rid your body of "love handles" by stretching and strengthening your waistline as well as improve balance

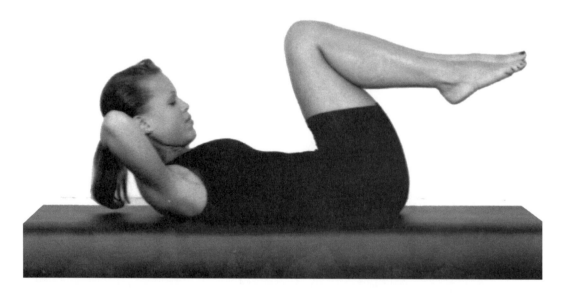

1. Lie on your back and bend your knees into your chest. Place your hands behind your head and keep the elbows open. Lift your shoulders off the mat and bring your chin towards your chest.

Moore College of Art president Barbara G. Price

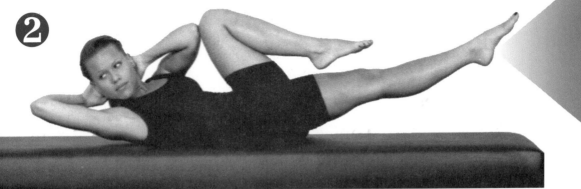

2. Bend your right knee into your chest while your left leg reaches out at an angle. Maintain a flat back, while working at the abdominals. Diagonally, bring the left elbow to the right knee. The right side of your body and your right elbow should twist behind you. Hold the position.

3. Switch to the opposite side. Focus on the stretching behind you. Repeat 5-10 times.

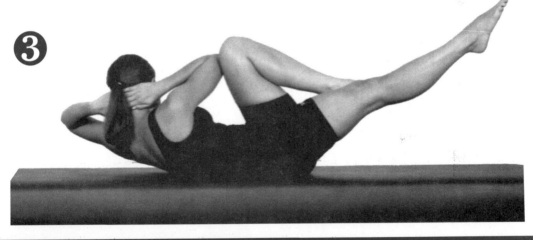

Focus Points

The most important part of this exercise is the twisting and reaching back. Slow down the tempo and hold the twist!

Make sure your shoulders and elbows stay off the mat to work deeper in the abdominals.

Exercise 9
Spine Stretch Forward

To stretch your spine and hamstrings as well as empty the air out of your lungs

①

②

1. Sit with your legs straight and open slightly wider than shoulder width. Extend your arms straight out at shoulder height.

2. Inhale and stretch your spine upwards moving from the head down. with your chin towards your chest, begin roll down and forward.

③

3. Keep your stomach muscles in and form a "C" with your lower back. Reach forward with a sliding motion. As the body stretches forward and down keep the hip bones over the tailbone. Pull the stomach in tight and exhale.

The Pilates® Method

"A soft fitness regime [i.e., The Pilates Method] can produce a hard body."

Investor's Business Daily

THE MAT

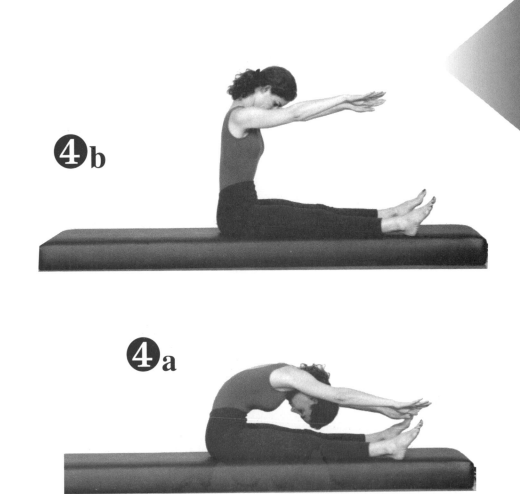

❹b

❹a

4a,b. On the inhalation, initiate from the navel and roll back up. Squeeze the buttocks, sit up tall and exhale as seen in Step 1. Repeat 3 times and try to reach further down and deeper into the spine with each repetition. Return to starting position.

Focus Points

Keep the abdominal wall drawn in and your chin pressed firmly against your chest. Concentrate on breathing into the lower spine.

This is a stretch "into" your spine. Open feet one inch past the width of your shoulders.

For a more challenging stretch, begin Step 1 with the feet flexed at a 90 degree angle and the toes pointing toward the ceiling.

49

Exercise 10
Open Leg Rocker

GOAL

To stretch your legs and arms and build up the spine

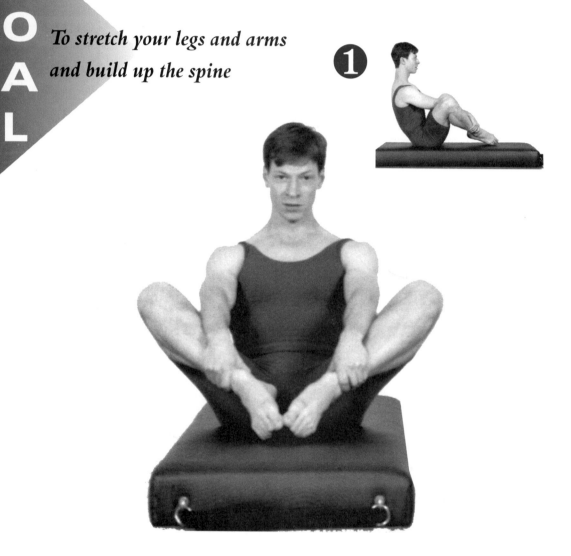

1. Balancing on your buttocks, lightly hold onto your ankles (or toes) as you simultaneously bend both legs towards you.

2a. Straighten both legs upward and **2b.** open to shoulder width while keeping the abdomen "drawn in." Inhale.

3. Keeping hold of your ankles, bring your feet down and in toward you. Repeat 6 times.

"People won't understand the brilliance of my work for 50 years."

Joseph H. Pilates, about 50 years ago

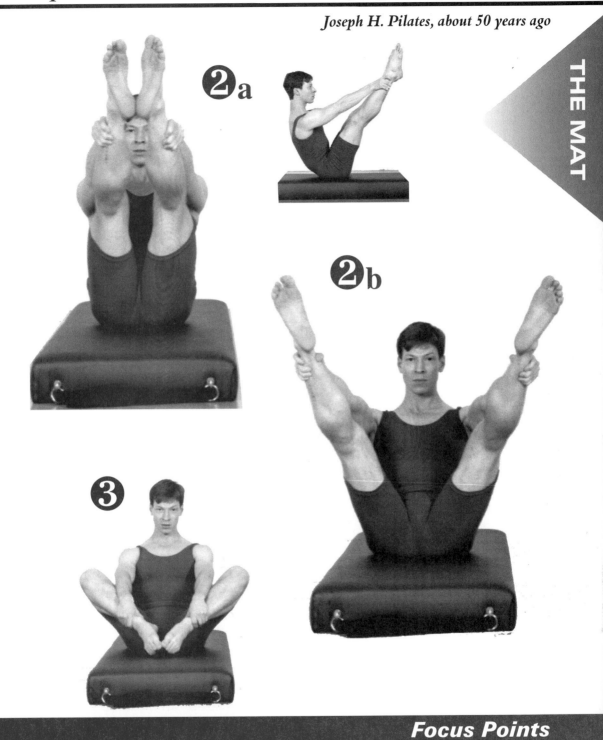

THE MAT

Focus Points

Once you have mastered the balance of this exercise, add a back roll to it. Exhale and roll back, keeping your chin firmly against your chest and your arms and legs straight. Inhale and roll back up, pivoting on the base of your spine. Do not roll down further than you can roll back up.

For people with stiff backs, try this exercise by holding onto extension straps on your feet or around your ankles.

51

Exercise 11
The Saw

A breathing exercise to trim your waist line and stretch your hamstrings

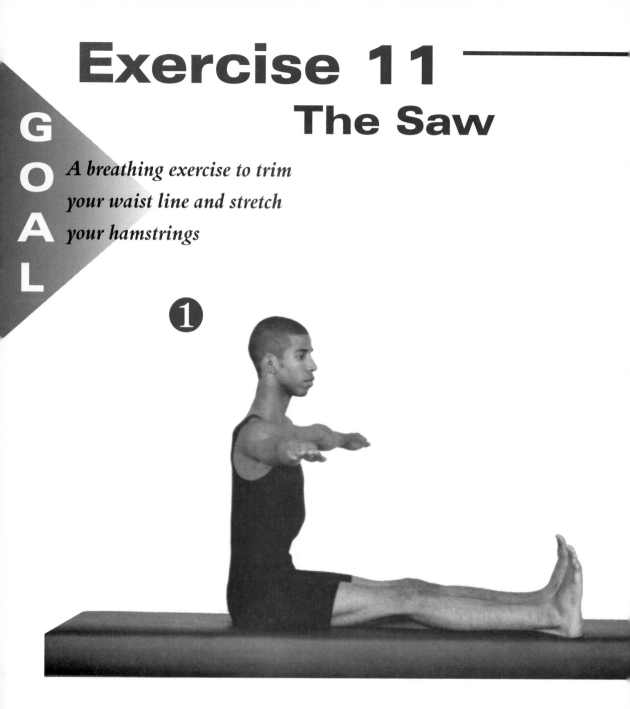

①

1. Sit up tall with your legs slightly wider than hip width apart. Extend the arms open to the sides. Draw the abdomen in.

"It immediately made me taller, leaner and stronger."

Pilates student Margaret Klugman

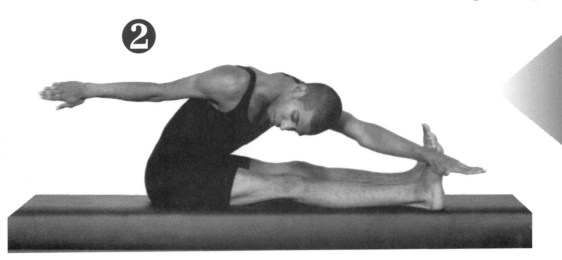

2. Drop the left arm and roll with your spine down over the right leg. Exhaling slowly, twist the spine to the right with your waist (not the pelvis). Squeeze the buttocks. With your little finger on your left hand passing the little toe of your right foot, perform 3 "saw-like" pulses, stretching the waist. Complete the exhalation. Initiating from the navel, roll up and return to the center.

3. Repeat to the left side. Do 4 sets.

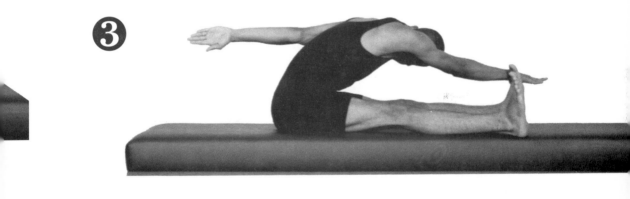

Focus Points

Open feet one inch past the width of your shoulders.

Twist your body before bending forward. Keep both hips squared and sit firmly into the mat. Reach into the opposite side of your waist as you reach with the forward arm.

Drop your back arm as your body twists to avoid injuring your shoulder.

Exercise 12
The Neck Roll

To release the tension from
your neck and shoulders

①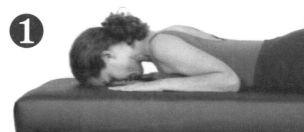

1. Lie on your stomach with your
hands placed on the mat under
your shoulders. Bring your legs
together.

②

2. On the inhalation and working
your back muscles, lift your
head and chest. Exhaling, continue the backbend until you
are fully upright.

③a

3a. Keeping your shoulders
down, gently roll your
head towards your
right shoulder,

The Pilates® Method

"Unlike aerobics, it's an overall feeling of well-being."

Devra Barratt Thompson, Pilates student

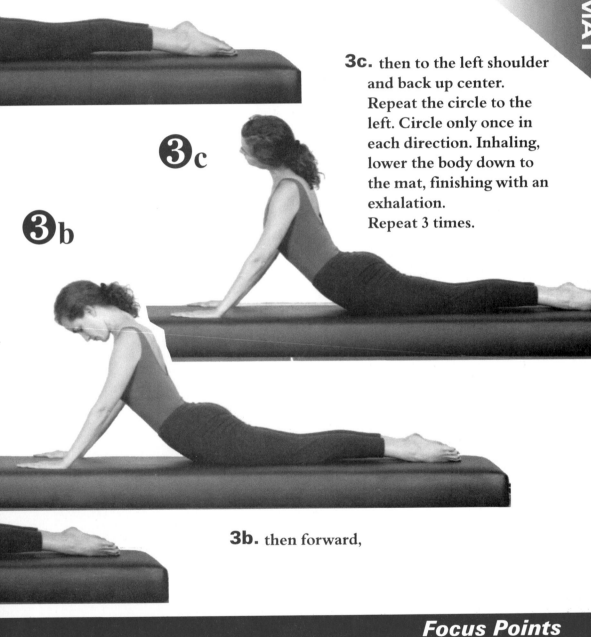

3c. then to the left shoulder and back up center. Repeat the circle to the left. Circle only once in each direction. Inhaling, lower the body down to the mat, finishing with an exhalation. Repeat 3 times.

3b. then forward,

Focus Points

CAUTION: Backbends should be done only by those who have a strong degree of Powerhouse control.

Keep your legs together as if they were one. Use the Powerhouse to arch the back as much as possible.

Exercise 13
Single Leg Kicks

To stretch your thighs, tighten your pectoral muscles and lift your biceps and triceps

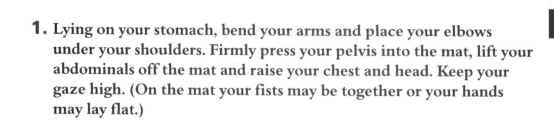

①

1. Lying on your stomach, bend your arms and place your elbows under your shoulders. Firmly press your pelvis into the mat, lift your abdominals off the mat and raise your chest and head. Keep your gaze high. (On the mat your fists may be together or your hands may lay flat.)

The Pilates® Method

Stuttgart Pilates instructor Ursula Bischoff-Musshake

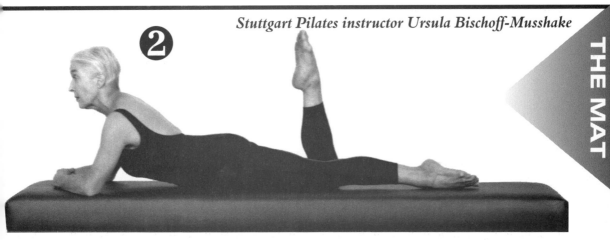

2. Kick your right heel with a double beat to the buttocks as the other leg stretches straight out on the mat. Do not allow your hips to lift.

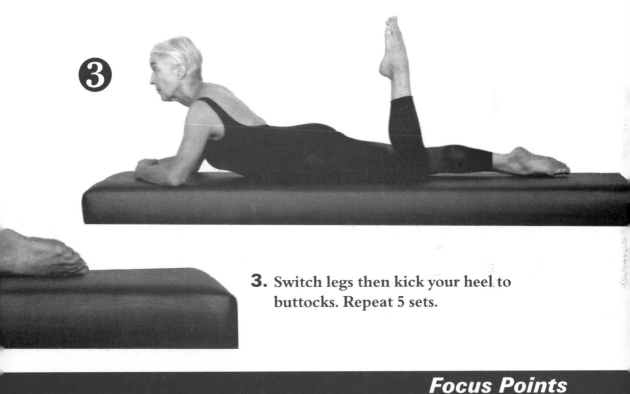

3. Switch legs then kick your heel to buttocks. Repeat 5 sets.

Focus Points

To prevent "sinking" into the lower back, lift the navel into the spine.

Maintain a long neck while looking up. Do not crunch your neck into your shoulders.

For people with bad knees, instead of kicking use an extra strap around your foot and slowly bend your knee as much as possible.

Exercise 14
Neck Pull

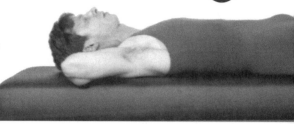

G O A L

To strengthen your Powerhouse, articulate your spine and stretch your hamstrings

①

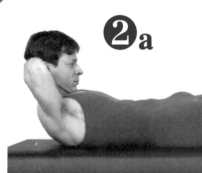

②a

1. Lie flat on your back, legs straight and hip width apart with the feet relaxed. Bring your stomach muscles in and place your hands behind your head.

②b

③

2a,b. Inhale slowly as you roll your chin up to your chest. Keep your elbows open and your abdomen drawn in throughout.

3. Exhale slowly. "Bow" the spine forward, pressing the legs firmly against the mat. Exhale completely as your bend your body forward over.

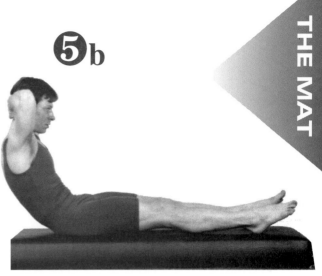

⑤b

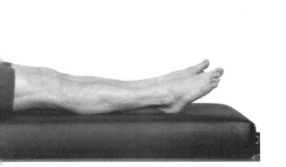

5a,b. Exhaling slowly, bring your stomach muscles in and squeeze the buttocks. Roll back down to the mat one vertebrae at a time. Roll "out" first, focusing on the lower back return to starting position. Repeat 5 times.

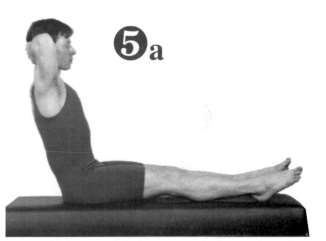

⑤a

④

4. Initiating from the navel, inhale while you roll up tall to a sitting position with a straight back.

Focus Points

If you are having difficulty rolling up, either place your feet underneath a strap or have a partner or trainer hold your feet for resistance.

A partner or trainer can add an extra stretch by opening your back and shoulder girdle from behind as you sit tall before rolling down.

Exercise 15 ———
Side-Kicks

To stretch your legs and hips as well as control your Powerhouse and upper body

1

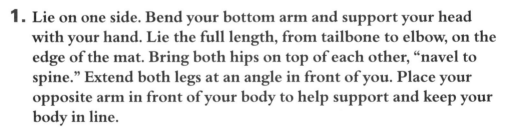

1. Lie on one side. Bend your bottom arm and support your head with your hand. Lie the full length, from tailbone to elbow, on the edge of the mat. Bring both hips on top of each other, "navel to spine." Extend both legs at an angle in front of you. Place your opposite arm in front of your body to help support and keep your body in line.

2. Lift the top leg to hip height. Keep the leg long and soft.

3. Inhaling slowly, swing the leg forward as far up as possible while maintaining the correct placement. Perform 2 pulses.

4. Exhaling slowly, swing the leg backward, reaching it as far behind the body as you can without shifting in the ribcage or in hip placement. Repeat a maximum of 10 times on each side.

"His methods ... are tuned so that the sum of all exercises balance out the entire musculature and the joints are relieved of much strain."

Stuttgart Pilates instructor Ursula Bischoff-Musshake

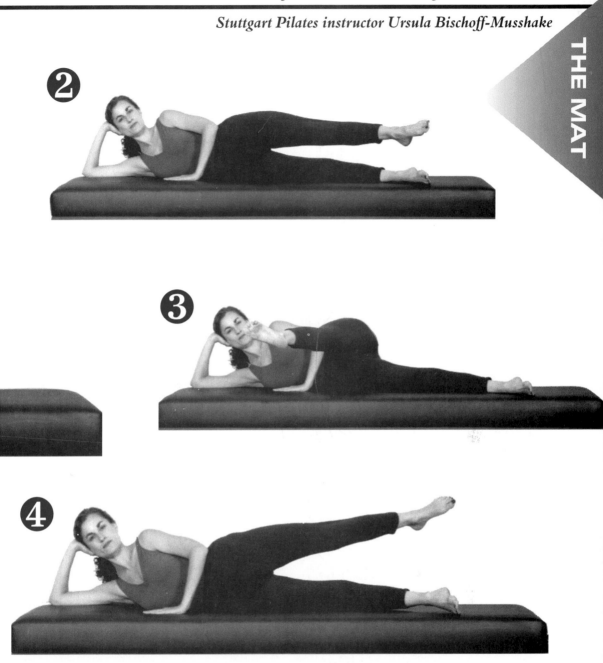

Focus Points

Keep the entire body firmly placed. Only the leg moves freely, swinging like a pendulum. Work with long, soft pointed legs. Keep swinging leg at an even height.

If you cannot prevent shifting in your body, limit your range of movement.

Keep the feet relaxed. For most people, avoid a pointing or flexing motion that will only work the lower leg. This exercise works the upper leg.

61

Exercise 16
Side Kick Series:
Up and Down

To stretch your inner and outer thighs

①

1. Lie on your side propped up by your elbow. Place both legs at an angle in front of your body.

②

2. Lift the top leg straight up to the side. Inhale.

The Pilates® Method

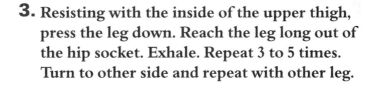

③

3. Resisting with the inside of the upper thigh,
press the leg down. Reach the leg long out of
the hip socket. Exhale. Repeat 3 to 5 times.
Turn to other side and repeat with other leg.

Focus Points

Make sure that as you lift your leg up you do not roll your hips forward or
backward. A partner or trainer can stand behind you and gently press
the hip in place.

Exercise 17
Side Kick Series: Small Circles

To stretch your inner and outer thighs

1. Begin in the same position as for the the Up-Down. (See Exercise 16.)

2. Keep your top leg at the height of your bottom heel.

3. Perform vigorous small circles as if you were drawing them with your toes. Do 5 to the front then 5 to the back. Repeat on the other leg.

"It's never boring. It's really challenging and fun."

Pilates student Margaret Klugman

THE MAT

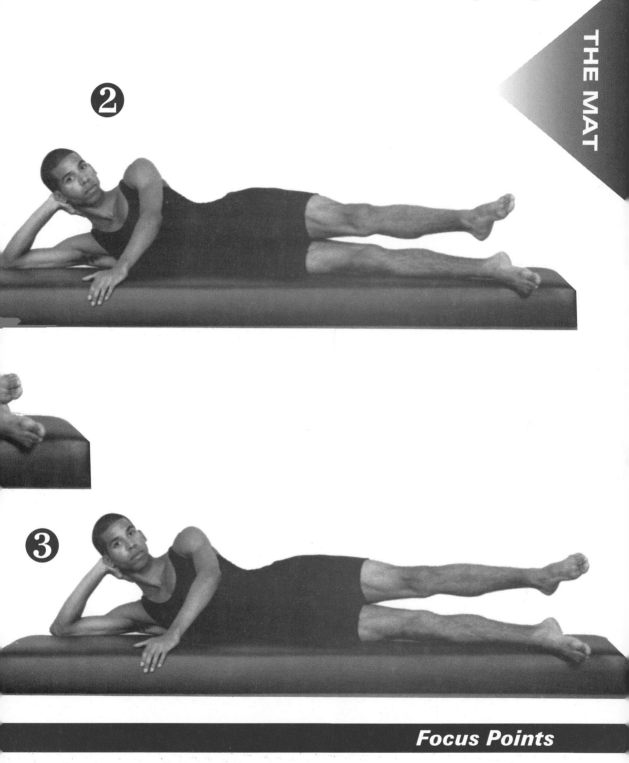

2

3

Focus Points

The rhythm is vigorous with the accent forward.

Lengthen the leg out of the hip.

Exercise 18
Teaser 1

A Powerhouse technique for balance and control. Develops proper breathing techniques

❶

❷

1. Lie flat on your back with your arms resting on the mat and stretched straight overhead. Put your knees into your chest.

2. Extend your legs out to a 45 degree angle to the mat. Bring your stomach muscles in and maintain a flat back.

❸a

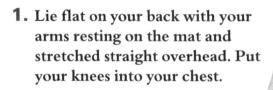

The Pilates® Method

"The exercises release so much from you that some people have ended up crying."

Brook Siler, Pilates Trainer

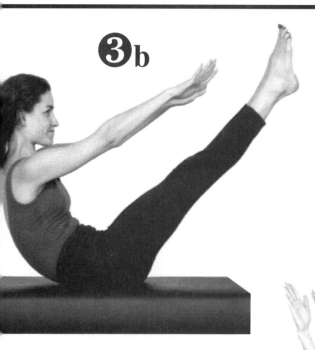

3b

④

3a., 3b. Initiating from the Powerhouse, roll into a V-position with your arms pointing to your toes. Keep your legs on the same level. Inhale.

4. Exhale, bring your arms up to your ears and with control roll down to the mat.

Note: Advanced step: Stay in the up position and lift your arms straight up and back by your ears. Reach for the wall behind you. This really works the waistline.

Focus Points

If you have weak abdominal control and cannot do the exercise as described, try the following variation:

Have a partner or trainer stand in front of you and place your feet on their thighs, making sure your legs are not higher than 45 degrees off the mat. With help, roll up while they hold your hand. Roll down only halfway the first three times, then roll all the way down. On the way down your partner or trainer should use their Powerhouse to resist you so they don't injure their back.

Exercise 19 ——
Teaser 2

To develop proper breathing, balance and control

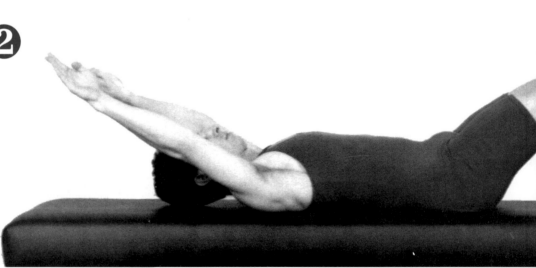

1. Lie flat on your back with your knees bent to your chest and your lower legs parallel to the mat.

2. Extend your legs so they are at a 45 degree angle from the mat, keeping a flat back firmly connected to the mat.

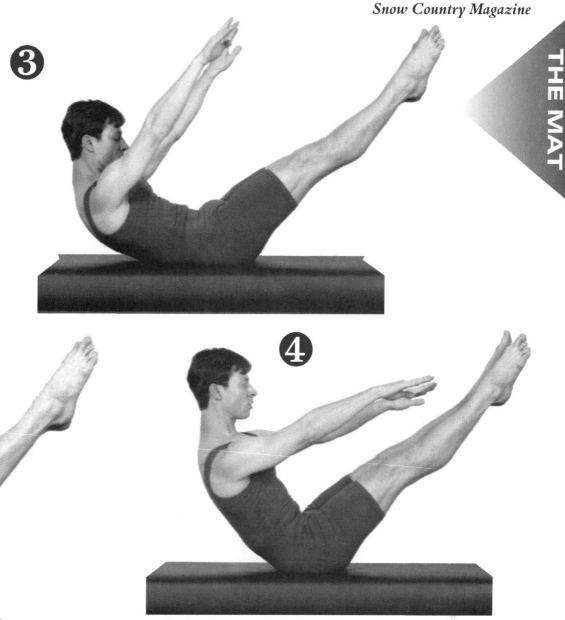

3. Initiating from the Powerhouse, roll up and reach your hands towards your toes.

4. Keep the upper body still and at a constant angle while lowering and raising your legs. Repeat 3 to 5 times. With control, slowly roll down to the mat.

Focus Points

Keep the range of leg movement small. They only go as far down as they can come back up. Keep the accent on the up.

While working the legs with a strong Powerhouse, hold the upper body in a stable position.

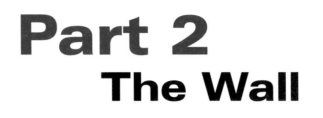

Part 2
The Wall

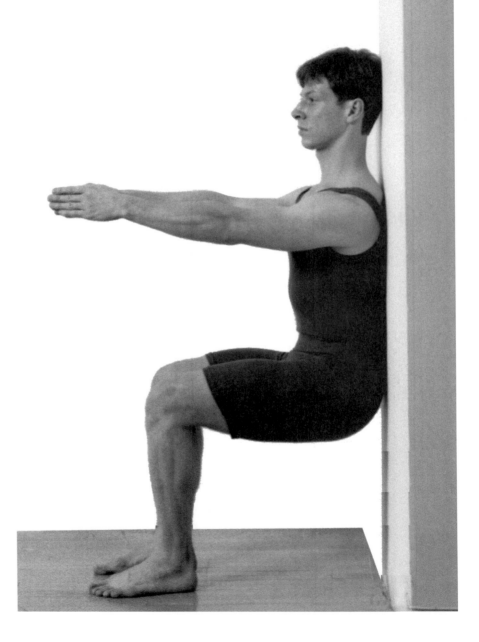

The Wall is the only Pilates exercise which requires no special equipment. It can be performed anywhere at anytime whether at home or work. The Wall works each vertebra of the spine, while expanding the lungs, stretching the muscles, draining tension from the neck and shoulders and strengthening the thighs

Objectives:

Work the spine
Expand the lungs
Stretch the muscles
Drain tension from the upper body
Strengthen the thighs

Exercise 20
The Roll Down

To drain tension from the neck and shoulders and develop awareness of spine and Powerhouse

1a. Start with your head and back against the wall. **1b.** Drop your head forward and let its weight slowly "peel" your spine off the wall.

1c. Work one vertebra at a time, keeping your stomach muscles in throughout.

The Pilates® Method

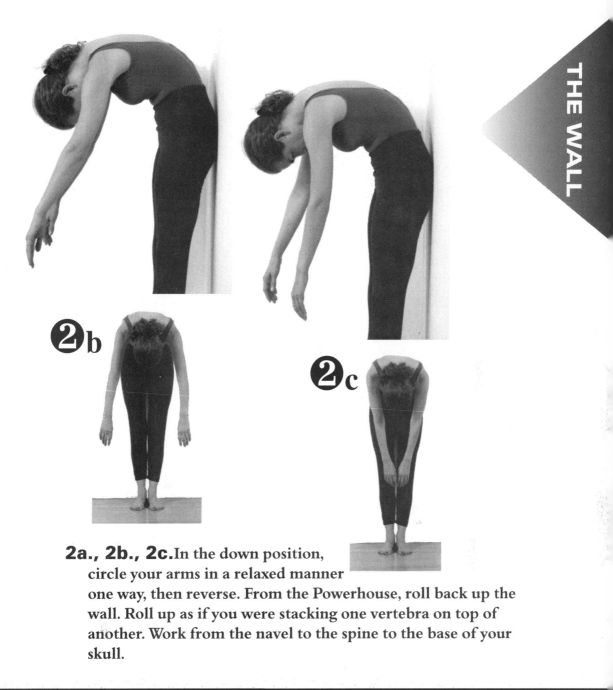

THE WALL

2a., 2b., 2c. In the down position, circle your arms in a relaxed manner one way, then reverse. From the Powerhouse, roll back up the wall. Roll up as if you were stacking one vertebra on top of another. Work from the navel to the spine to the base of your skull.

Focus Points

Stiff people will roll as far down as they can to stretch.

Holding weights is optional.

Exercise 21
Sitting on the Chair

Strengthen and
stretch the thighs

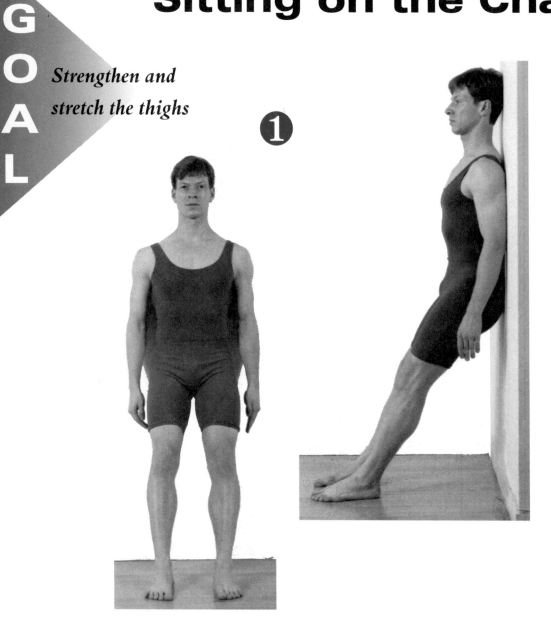

1 Lean your body flat against the wall. Turn your feet parallel to each other and perpendicular to the wall, hip width apart and place them some distance from the wall.

2. Bending the knees, slide the spine along the wall lowering the upper body as if you were sitting in an invisible chair. Do not go lower than right angle in the knees. Slide up.

The Pilates® Method

> *"By exercising your stomach muscles you wring out the body, you don't catch colds, you don't get cancer, you don't get hernias"*

Joseph H. Pilates, 1962

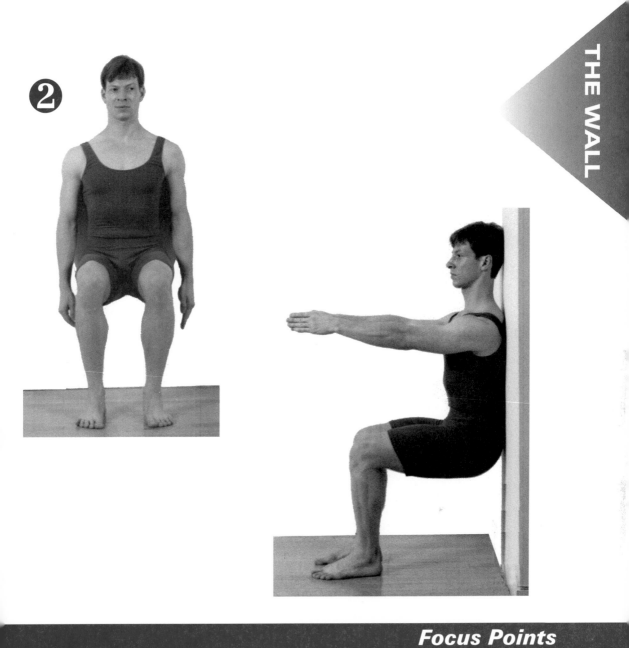

Focus Points

If you cannot maintain the posture as shown then bring your head away from the wall.

Simultaneously lifting your forearms forward or overhead is more challenging.

Pull navel to spine. Hold your back flat against the wall.

Part 3
Wall Springs
(The Cadillac)

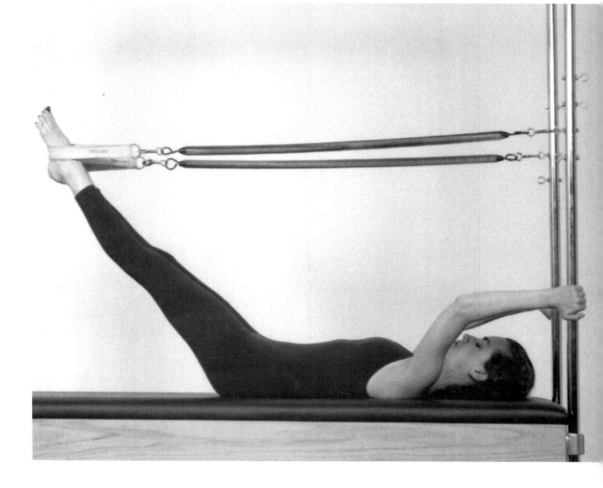

Developed by Joseph H. Pilates for hospital patients, Springs are used to provide resistance exercises, mainly to stretch and articulate and stabilize the spine. For home use, springs and hooks can be purchased to simulate the Cadillac by using any door frame.

CAUTION: Some spring exercises can be difficult for beginners to control. We recommend working with a partner or with a certified Pilates instructor. If you have bad knees avoid the leg spring exercises.

Objectives:

Opening up and articulating the spine
Stretch the sides
Strengthen the Powerhouse, legs, arms
        and spinal column
Slimming the thighs
Stretch and strengthen the hips,
        waistline, neck, back and legs
Improve the breathing
Enhance the body's coordination
Increase flexibility in the shoulders
Strengthen the upper body
Lengthen the upper arms
Correct body alignment
Massage the entire body and
        internal organs

SUBSTITUTION: Springs and mounting hooks can be purchased from the Pilates Studio®. A mat or soft carpet is necessary for these exercises.

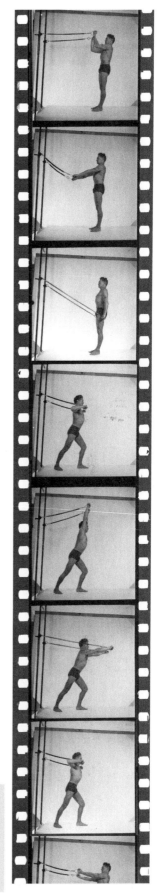

Exercise 22
Rolling Back

GOAL

Articulate the full spine

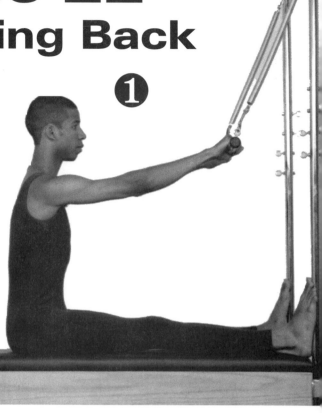

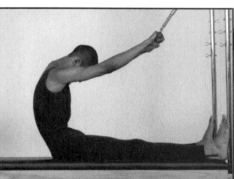

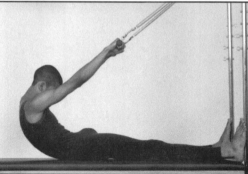

1. Sit on the floor with the soles of your feet against the door frame, holding onto the bar.

2. Let your head drop to your chest. Push your heels into the door frame.

3. Then using the Powerhouse, slowly roll down one vertebra at a time.

The Pilates® Method

"Not only is the body rejuvenated, but the mental and spiritual refreshment is beyond calculation."

Dancer Ruth S. Denis

4. Focus on the first 5 vertebrae, then take your time working through the vertebrae of the rib cage, then opening your shoulders and collarbones, and,

5. finally resting your head and lengthening your neck.

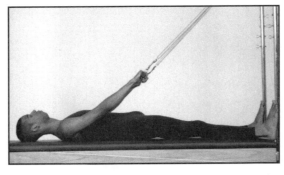

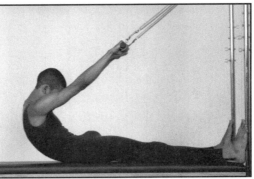

6. Bring your chin back onto your chest and slowly roll your way up again, one vertebra at a time. Repeat 3 times.

Focus Points

This exercise should be performed with straight legs. However, If you have trouble articulating your spine you may slightly bend your knees.

With very stiff backs, hold for a moment in the stiffest region to work those vertebrae.

79

Exercise 23
Leg Circles

Controlling the lower back, strengthening the legs and slimming the thighs

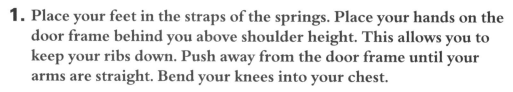

1. Place your feet in the straps of the springs. Place your hands on the door frame behind you above shoulder height. This allows you to keep your ribs down. Push away from the door frame until your arms are straight. Bend your knees into your chest.

2. Extend your legs out in front of your hips, but never to a 90 degree angle up.

3. Then open your legs as wide as you can while still maintaining control.

The Pilates® Method

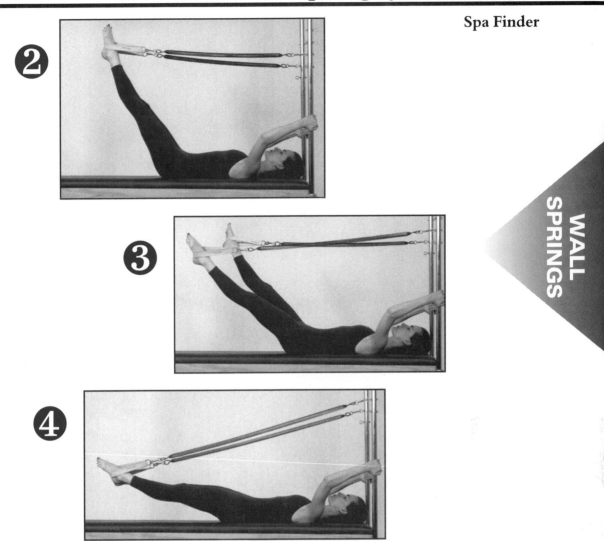

WALL SPRINGS

4. Pull your legs down. Use the Powerhouse to keep your back on the mat. Working from the inside of your thighs, close your legs and then, with control, bring your legs back up. Focus on working symmetrically and drawing circles with your legs. Make sure you maintain the tension evenly in the springs. Repeat 5-10 times, then reverse the circles.

Focus Points

Do not attempt this exercise if you have bad knees.

Work slowly and precisely in the beginning. Always start small. Later you can go as wide as you can control.

Walking

To develop your back as well as working your glutes and inner and outer thighs

❶

1. Lie on the floor with your feet placed into the straps, knees bent into the chest. This starting position is the same as Leg Circles.

The Pilates® Method

"I've lost inches, I have more command of my physical instrument and I've become highly focused and centered ."

Opera soprano Roberta Prada

②a

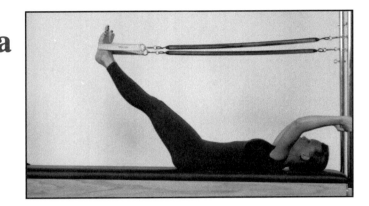

2a. Extend your legs out. **2b.**Walk your legs down with even steps pulling the springs. Walk a maximum of eight steps down. Walk back up with the same eight steps, using the Powerhouse to control back placement. Keep walking. Do three sets of eight up and down.

WALL SPRINGS

②b

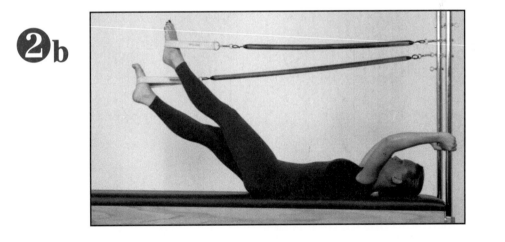

Focus Points

Go only as far down as you can maintain your back on the floor.

Make sure you work the springs with control, with legs and hips even. Maintain tension on the springs at all times.

In between exercises in this series, relax your arms down alongside the body and bend the knees into the chest.

Exercise 25
Beats

To develop your lower back and inner leg muscles

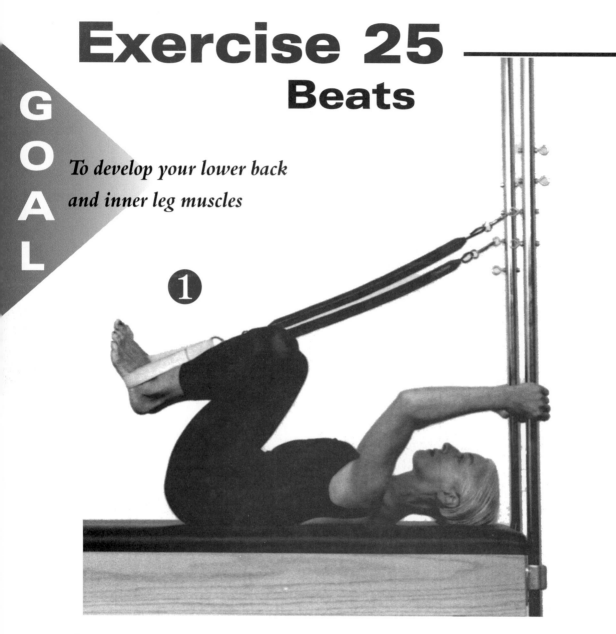

1. The starting position is the same as Leg Circles and Walking.

2. Extend the legs outward. With rapid movements, beat the inner thighs in and out for 8-10 repetitions. Make the beats vigorous. Repeat 3 sets.

3. Advanced step: vary the angle at which you extend your legs — the lower you reach the more challenging the exercise becomes. Bring feet to shoulder width. Make sure the Powerhouse keeps your back flat and your hips square.

4. Return to starting position.

"It sort of undoes everything that you've done to your body through the course of the day."

Jane Moses, interim director, Pennsylvania Ballet

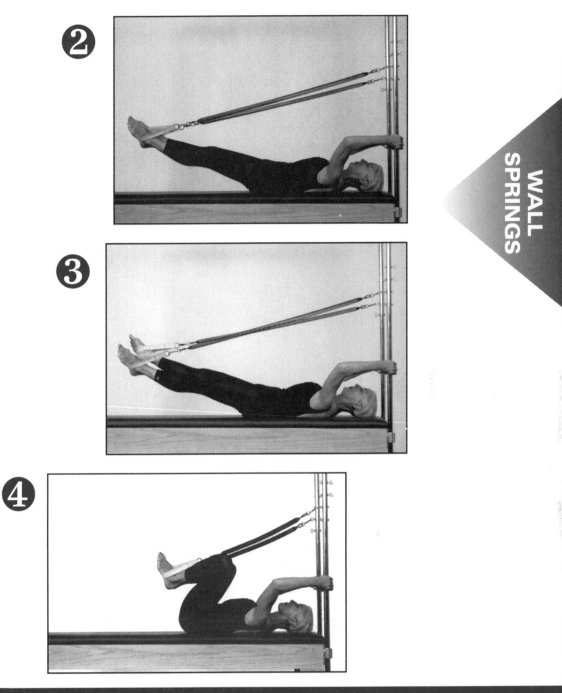

Focus Points

As you become more skilled and limber keep your arms straight instead of bent as shown in the photos.

Exercise 26
Rond de Jambe

To work your inner and outer thighs and to reshape and firm up your buttocks and lower back

①

1. Starting position is the same as Leg Circles (See Exercise 23).

The Pilates® Method

"There's definitely that kind of yoga feeling afterwards."

Jane Moses

a

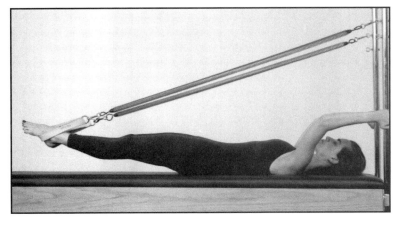

2a,b. Extend your legs to a 30 degree angle from the floor. Bring your feet to shoulder width. With legs outstretched make small "springy" circles within your hip sockets for 5 repetitions. Reverse the direction of the circles. Repeat for 3 sets.

b

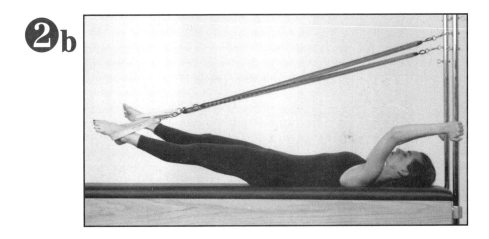

WALL SPRINGS

Focus Points

This is a variation designed for dancers and advanced Pilates students.

Make sure the Powerhouse holds the back to the mat.

Work the legs and springs level and evenly while circling.

Exercise 27
Chest Expansion

Upper body control, breathing, neck stretch

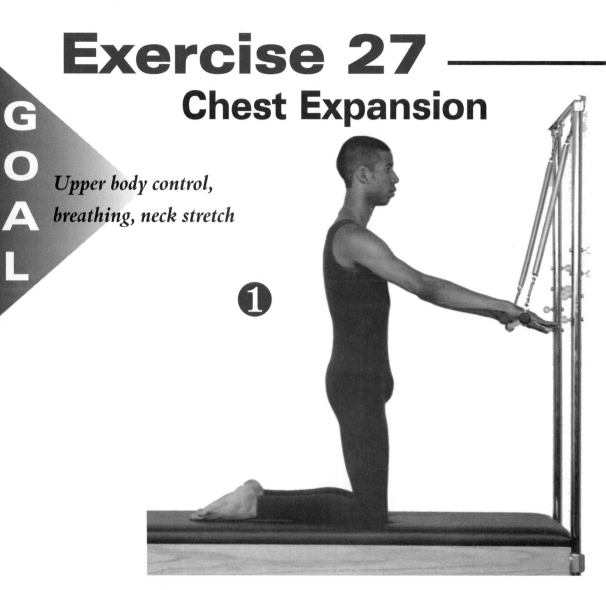

1

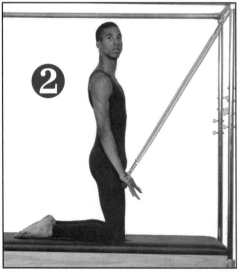

2

1. Kneel on the floor facing the door about one arm's length away. Your knees should be hip width apart. Place your hands on the bar or straps with your arms straight out.

2. Keeping your arms straight and inhaling, pull the bar or straps down to your thighs. While holding your breath and the bar, look down and to the right stretching the left side of your neck.

The Pilates® Method

*"I'm not concerned with body building.
I'm just trying to make people normal human beings."*

Joseph H. Pilates

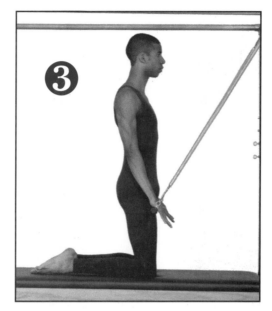

3. Return head to center.

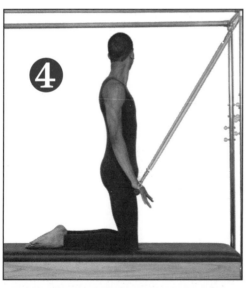

4. Then look to the left stretching to the right. Return to center. Exhale as you return the bar or straps up. Repeat reversing neck stretch order. Do 2 sets.

Focus Points

Make sure your body stays in one line. In other words, head over shoulders, over hips, over knees.

Make sure your shoulders don't shift when you look left and right.

Open the chest and pull your shoulders into your back before moving your arms.

This exercise can also be done in a standing position if kneeling causes discomfort.

Exercise 28
Bicycle

CAUTION: This exercise can cause injury if performed improperly.
We advise you to seek the aid of a trainer or instructor.

*Stretch and strengthen
the hip region*

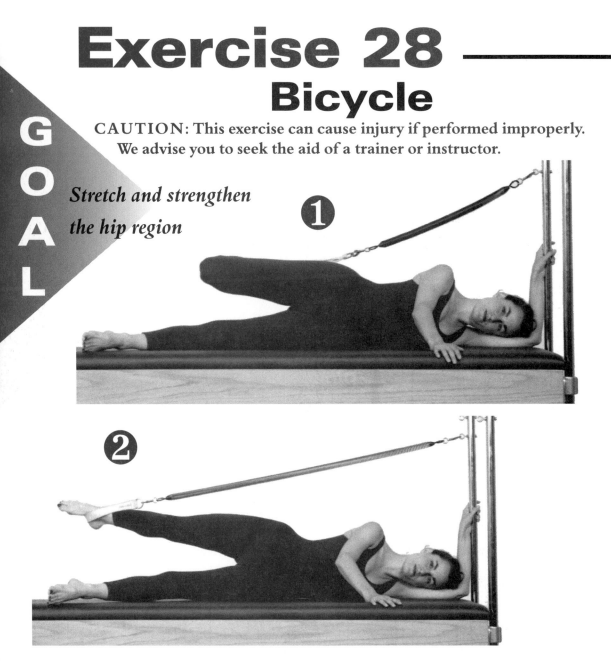

1. Lie on your side extending your legs away from the frame. Bend your lower arm at a right angle against the door. (An advanced variation has this arm straight for more stretch in the leg.) Place your top leg into the strap of the spring behind the body. Place your hips and shoulders perpendicular to the floor and keep them in that position throughout the exercise.

2. Bring your leg straight forward toward your head as high as possible while keeping hip height.

The Pilates® Method

> *"With a strong and stable torso, your limbs will move more freely, developing better balance and posture."*
>
> Bob Liekens, Pilates Studio supervising instructor

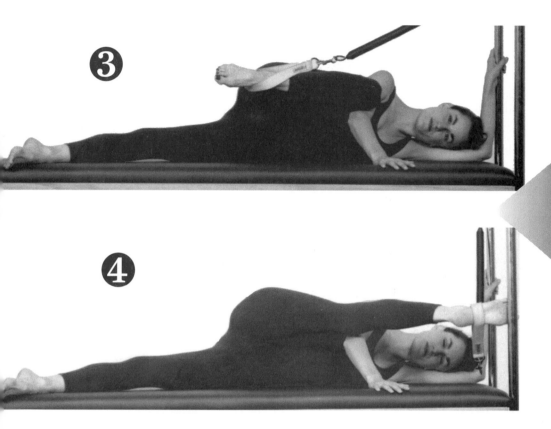

WALL SPRINGS

3. Bend your knee into your shoulder. Bring your knee to your bottom knee, opening the hip. Lift your heel back to your buttocks. Keeping your heel to your buttock lift your thigh back. Keep your knee in line with your hip.

4. Keep lifting your thigh as you straighten the leg. With a big circular movement, reach your leg back up to the door frame ready to start again. Repeat 2-3 times, then reverse. On the reverse, finish with the leg on the door frame. Reach up and take the strap off the foot. (For advanced students: roll into a split.)

Focus Points

This exercise is ideal for dancers who need more control.

This is a therapeutic exercise for sciatica.

The first few times you perform this exercise, a partner or trainer should stand behind you and guide your leg through its movements. The assistant should help maintain your leg at hip level. They should stretch your leg into your side and behind you. As you stretch back down, they should pull the leg gently, opening the hip.

Exercise 29
Boxing

Coordination, arm work,
body alignment

①

1. Hook two springs on the door frame. Stand facing away from the door in Pilates stance. With your Powerhouse in control and your body in a straight line, lie into the springs as shown. Bring your fists in line with your sternum.

The Pilates® Method

"Pilates is fun. Sessions zip by in no time at all."

Philadelphia Inquirer Magazine

2

2. Reach your right arm out and forward as if you were boxing. Return the right arm in.

WALL SPRINGS

3

3. Then alternate and work the left arm while controlling the spring. Repeat 8-10 movements.

Focus Points

Your body should remain still during this exercise. Keep your shoulders square. Only your arms move.

The arm movement initiates from the Powerhouse.

Keep tension on springs at all times.

Exercise 30 ———
Shaving the Head

Open the chest

1

1. Maintain the Pilates stance and keep your weight into the springs. Bend your arms behind the head, your hands forming a triangle at the base of the neck. Widen your chest and open your elbows well to the sides, behind the ears.

2. "Shave" the back of the head by extending your arms upward. Maintain your whole body in a long diagonal line forward.

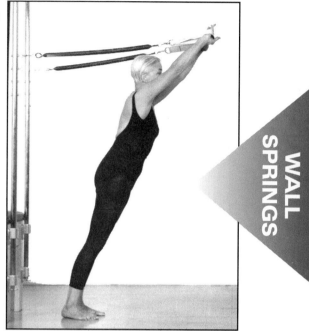

WALL SPRINGS

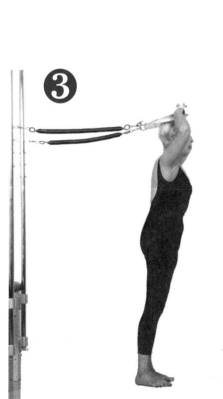

3. With control open your elbows sideways and return your hands to the base of your neck. Repeat 3 to 4 times.

Focus Points

Hold onto a firm Pilates stance. Work a long diagonal from your heels, through your spine, to the crown of your head then out to your finger tips.

Hold your elbows behind your ears, opening the chest. Keep your gaze up.

Exercise 31
The Hug

Work the chest and
shoulders, breathing

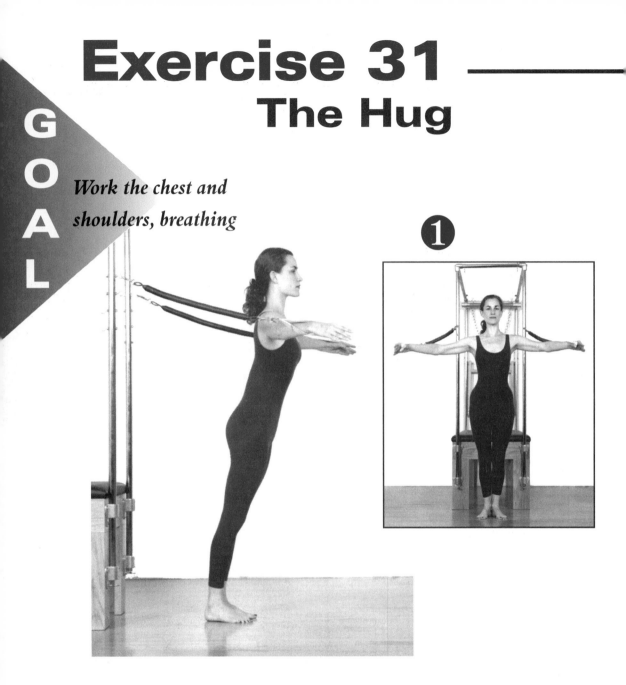

❶

1. Standing in a strong Pilates stance, lean the entire body forward, open your arms to the sides and keep them at shoulder height within your peripheral vision. Keep your elbows soft and lifted.

2. On the inhalation round both arms inward as if hugging a huge ball. Work the chest muscles.

3. On the exhalation, open the arms with resistance. Keep your body still as you open your arms. Repeat 2-3 times, then reverse the breathing.

> *"Six basic principles underlie the workout: proper breathing, control, concentration, centering, flowing movement and precision."*

Aliesa George-Jefferies, owner, Flinthills Physical Conditioning, Wichita, Kansas

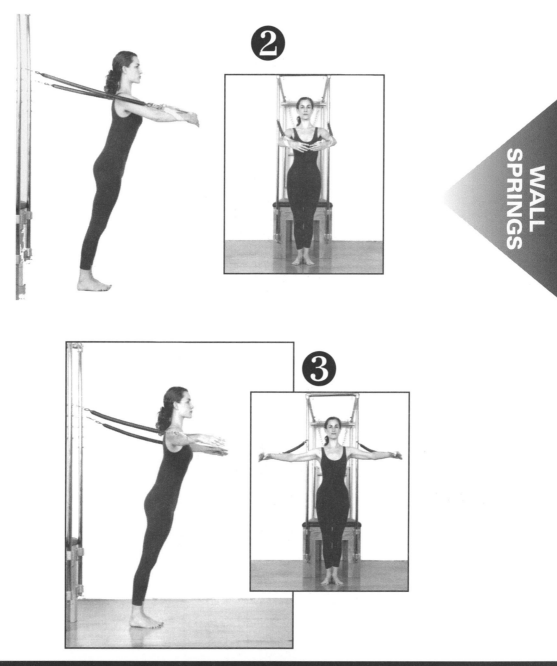

❷

❸

Focus Points

Watch that on the opening of your arms the springs do not pull you back. Keep your upper body in place.

Make your arms work from the Powerhouse, keeping the shoulders down into your back.

97

Exercise 32
Squat

Strengthen the quadriceps and stretch the back and hamstrings

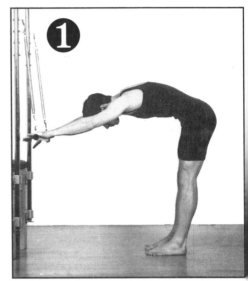

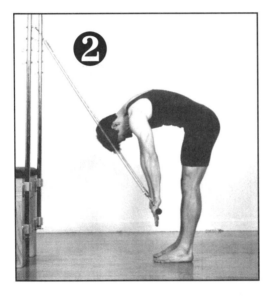

1. Hook the springs on the door frame at a little below shoulder height. Stand facing the door and hold onto the straps or bar. Stand far enough back to put tension in the springs and bend over through the Powerhouse.

2. Reach your arms down and toward your toes, working the springs. Keep your hips over your heels.

3. Return to the up position lifting your elbows in front of your shoulders. Bend your elbows to a 90 degree angle. Keep your fingers outstretched and your palms facing you.

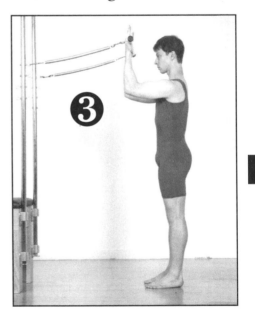

The Pilates® Method

"(Pilates) ... contours the body, reshapes the thighs, slims hips, and lifts the rear. You can go down a size."

Philadelphia Inquirer Magazine

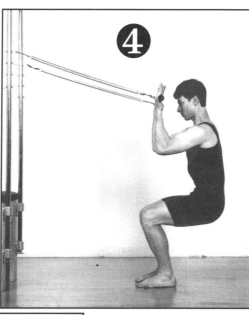

4. Bending your knees, lower yourself to a sitting position.

WALL SPRINGS

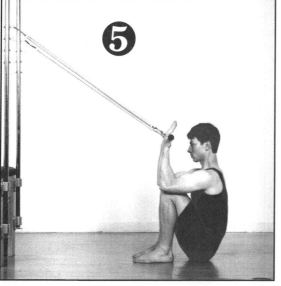

5. Sit on the floor as close to your heels as possible. Lift the points of your elbows forward and up, and by engaging the Powerhouse return to the position shown in step three. Keep the weight of your head forward. Repeat entire exercise 1 to 3 times.

Focus Points

Perform this exercise with caution if you have a bad back or weak knees. Take it slowly and bend only as far as you can without discomfort.

Make sure your energy stays up! Do not sink to the floor.

Do not use the shoulders to pull yourself up. The whole exercise is working the Powerhouse.

Advanced step: while squatting down, work with one leg up in front of you. Make sure your leg stays aligned with the center line of your body.

Part 4
The Magic Circle

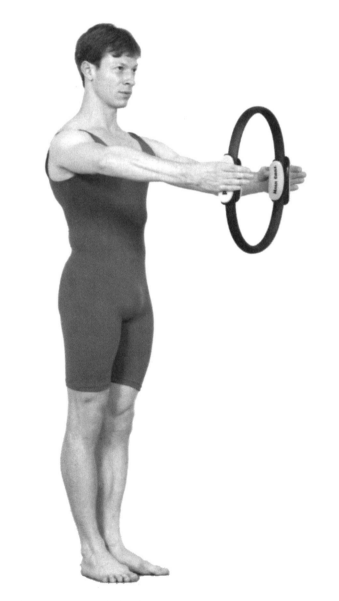

The Magic Circle, an inexpensive piece of Pilates equipment, provides low-stress resistance for gaining proper balance and posture, strengthening the arms and chest and reshaping the leg muscles and pelvis.

Objectives:

Helps to find the Powerhouse
Increase Powerhouse control
Gain balance, control and proper posture
Strengthen the muscles in the arms and chest
Strengthen and reshape the leg muscles
        and pelvis

SUBSTITUTION: You may use a ball 12" - 16" in diameter as a replacement for the Magic Circle.

Exercise 33 ———
Standing / Arms

For balance, control and proper posture. To strengthen muscles in your arms and chest

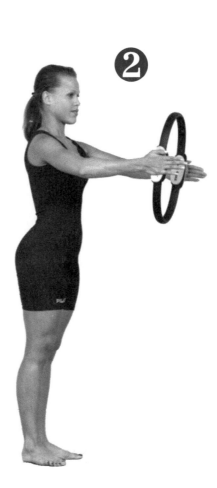

①

②

1. Stand in Pilates stance. Squeeze your buttocks and pull navel to spine. Take the Magic Circle between your hands keeping the fingers and wrists out-stretched. Lift your arms to shoulder height, keeping your elbows up.

2. Squeeze the Magic Circle and hold in place for 3 to 5 counts.

The Pilates® Method

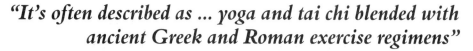

"It's often described as ... yoga and tai chi blended with ancient Greek and Roman exercise regimens"

Spa Magazine

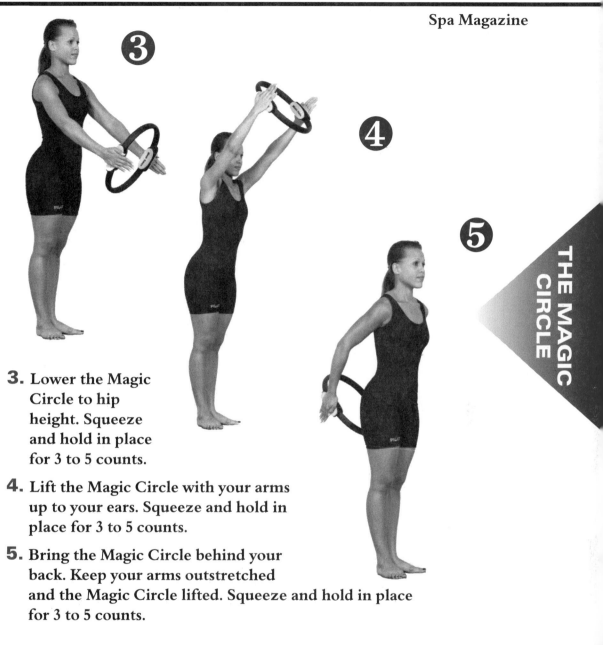

THE MAGIC CIRCLE

3. Lower the Magic Circle to hip height. Squeeze and hold in place for 3 to 5 counts.

4. Lift the Magic Circle with your arms up to your ears. Squeeze and hold in place for 3 to 5 counts.

5. Bring the Magic Circle behind your back. Keep your arms outstretched and the Magic Circle lifted. Squeeze and hold in place for 3 to 5 counts.

Focus Points

Advanced: When you get stronger, perform steps 2 through 5 by pulsing (squeeze in and out rapidly) for 10 vigorous repetitions.

Combine the movements. Start down while pulsing for 10 beats and gradually bring the Magic Circle up. Then lower for 10 beats.

Bring the Magic Circle to the side of your body. Place it on your hip. Bend your elbow but keep your wrist outstretched. Your fingers should point down. With the inside of your arm press the Magic Circle and hold for 3 counts.

Exercise 34 ———
Push Down

To strengthen and reshape your leg muscles and pelvis as well as increase Powerhouse control

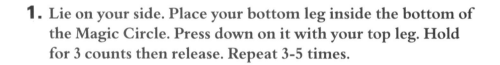

❶

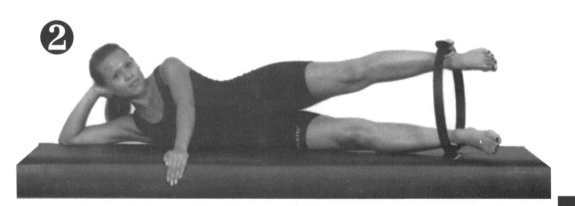

1. Lie on your side. Place your bottom leg inside the bottom of the Magic Circle. Press down on it with your top leg. Hold for 3 counts then release. Repeat 3-5 times.

❷

2. Place the top leg inside the top of the Magic Circle, push up and hold for 3 counts. Release and repeat.

❸

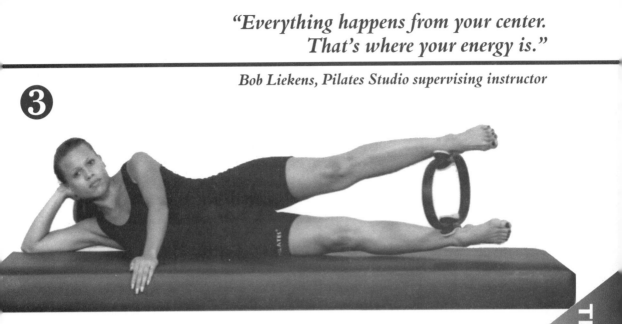

3. Place the Magic Circle between your legs. Lift both legs just off the floor then squeeze for three counts. Repeat.

THE MAGIC CIRCLE

❹

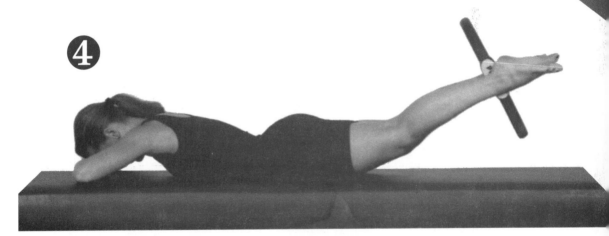

4. Turn to your stomach. Lift your thighs off the mat and squeeze with the inner thighs. Return to starting position. Roll over to your other hip and repeat.

Focus Points

The Magic Circle works with the Powerhouse in this exercise.

In Step 4, don't worry if you can't lift your legs as high as shown. Use this as a goal and only lift as high as you can.

Part 5
Small & Large Barrels
(Spine Corrector)

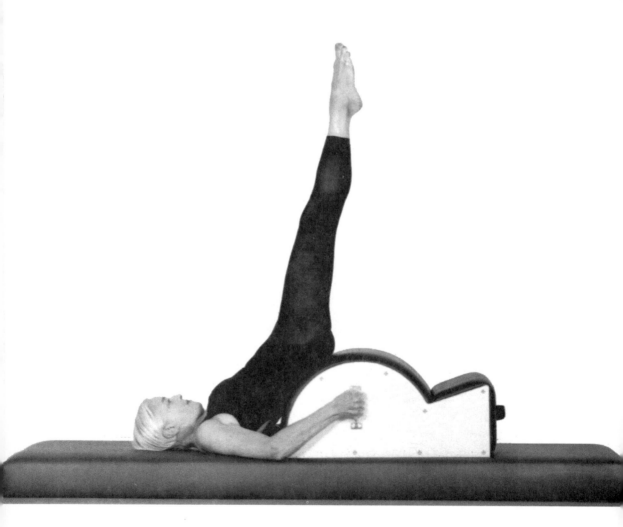

The Pilates® Method

The small and large Barrels used in the Pilates® Method enhance breathing, develop both the arms and legs, and work the spine to help correct posture and movement.

NOTE: Those with bad knees should work the Barrels instead of the leg exercises in the Wall Springs.

Objectives:

Stretch and align the spine

Enhance breathing

Stretch and strengthen upper back and neck

Open chest and lungs

Strengthen rotator cuff muscles

Lengthen thigh and calf muscles

Slim down bulky thighs

Strengthen inner and outer thighs

Massage lower back

Tone fleshy hips

Lengthen leg muscles

SUBSTITUTION: The Barrels can be substituted by using firm pillows, both small and large.

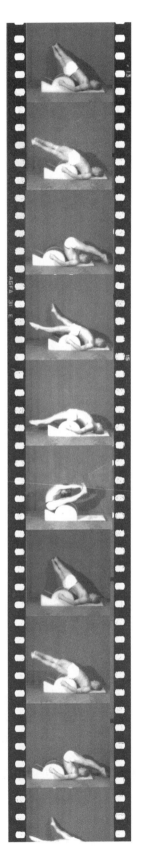

Exercise 35 ——
Arm Extension
(Small Barrel)

A breathing exercise designed to open your chest and lungs. Stretch your upper back and neck

1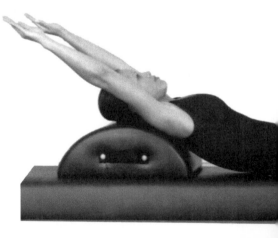

2

3

1. Lie with your upper back against the small Barrel or pillow. Place your head back with a long, relaxed neck. Extend your legs down into a Pilates stance. Your arms should be at your sides.

"Pilates can be adapted to people of every age and level of fitness, including pregnant women."

Spa Finder

2. Inhale and lift your arms straight towards the ceiling.

3. On the exhalation reach your arms back with 3 gentle pulses, gradually increasing the stretch. Keep your back to the Barrel or pillow.

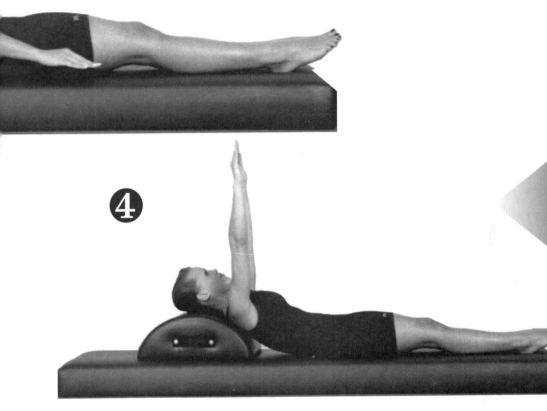

BARRELS

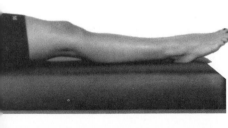

4. Inhale and lift your arms back up. Exhale and return your arms to your sides. Repeat 3 sets.

Focus Points

As you perform this exercise make certain the small of your back is firmly planted on the mat.

This exercise can be done with or without weights. A weighted bar can be used in the up and down stretches.

Exercise 36

Arm Circles
(Small Barrel)

A breathing exercise designed to open your chest and lungs. Stretch your upper back and neck

①

②

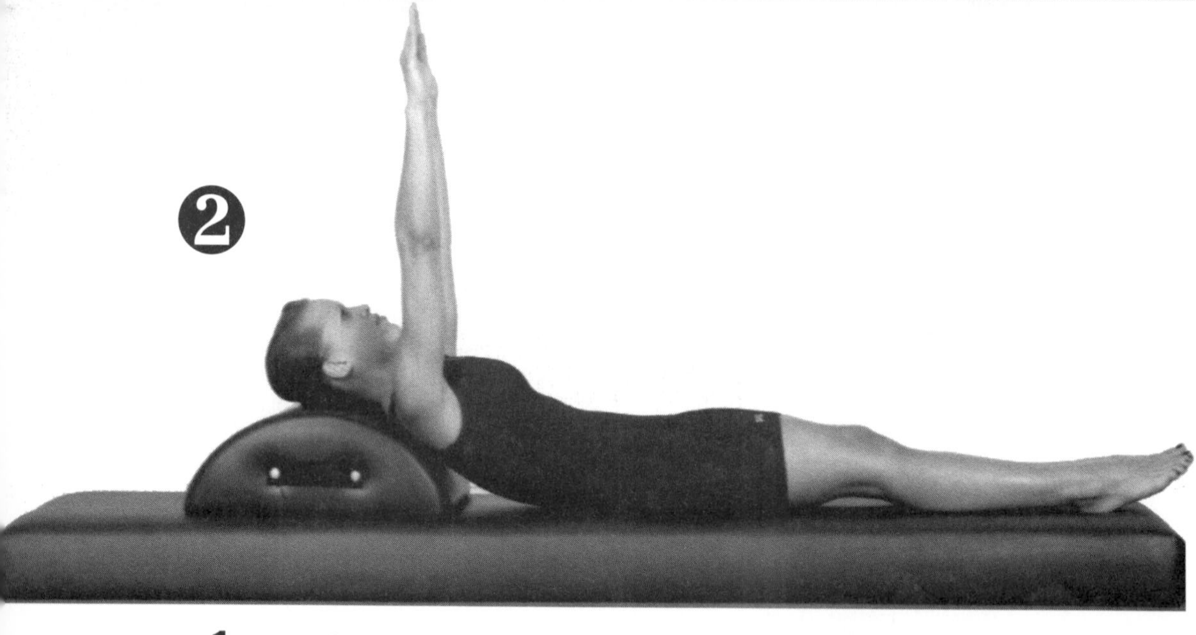

1. Use the same beginning position as Arm Extension as shown in previous exercise.

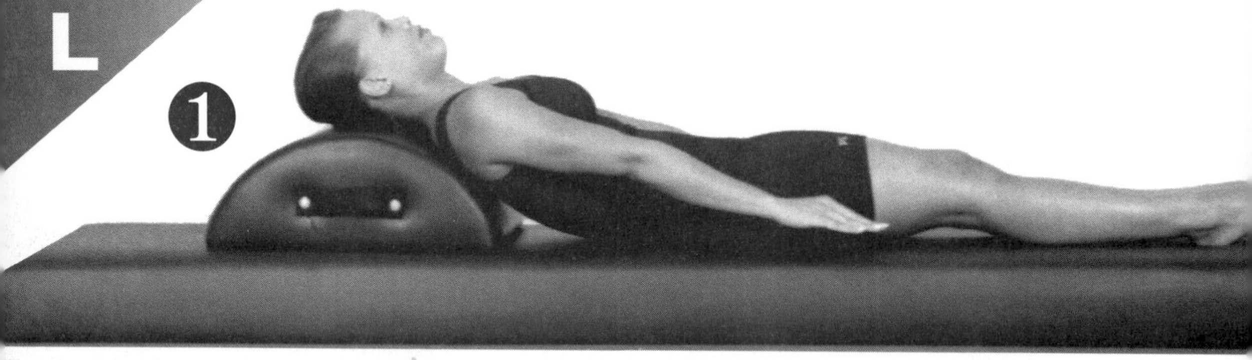

2. Inhale and lift your arms towards the ceiling.

3a,b,c. Circle 3 times in one direction, then reverse. When you can control the small circles, increase the diameter.

The Pilates® Method

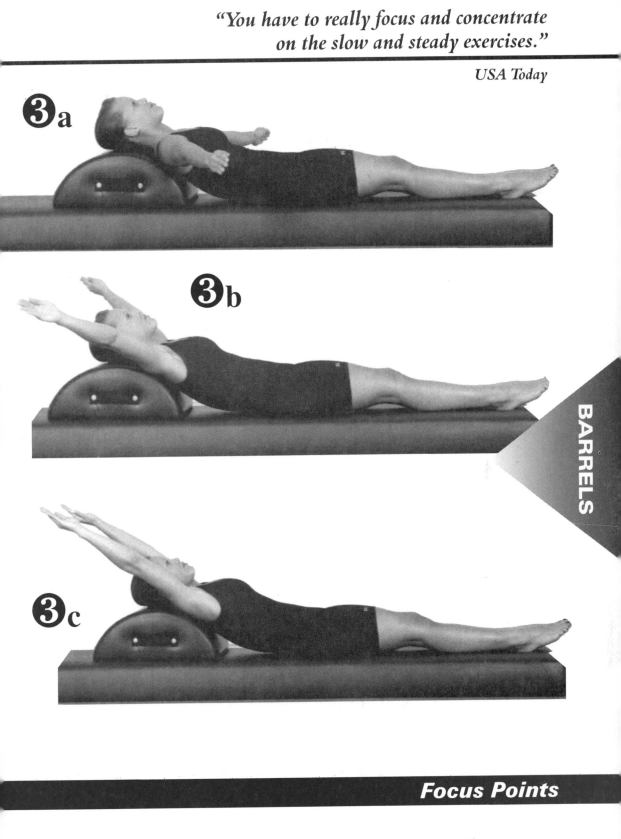

3a

3b

3c

BARRELS

Focus Points

After the initial series, to increase your stretch start higher up on the
Barrel or pillow and repeat the arm circles.

Exercise 37

Spine Corrector Arm Circles

To strengthen your rotator cuff muscles as well as your upper back and neck

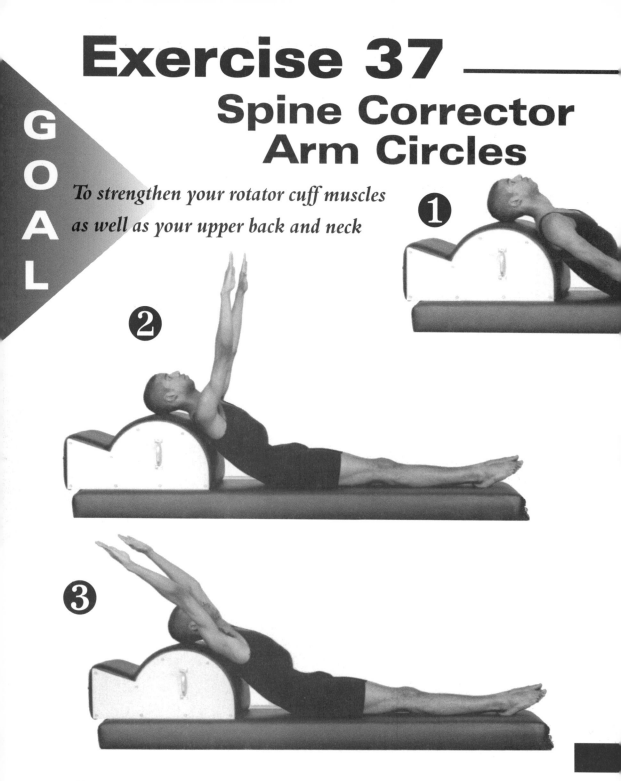

1. Sit on the mat with your upper back and head resting against the large Barrel or pillow. Your arms should be at your side.

2. Inhaling, lift your arms straight up to the ceiling.

3. Raise your arms in line with your ears.

The Pilates® Method

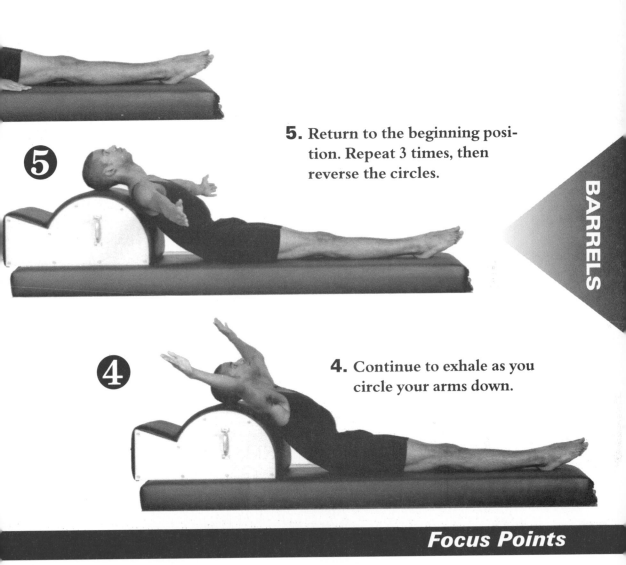

5. Return to the beginning position. Repeat 3 times, then reverse the circles.

4. Continue to exhale as you circle your arms down.

BARRELS

Focus Points

This exercise can be done with or without weights. If weights are used, 2 to 3 pounds are recommended.

Start with a slight arch in your upper back. Sit closer to the Barrel or pillow for a more intense stretch.

Introduce this exercise with an up/down movement and circle the arms later.

Add a cushion under your neck if you experience strain.

Exercise 38
Circles

To control the Powerhouse with support, while developing the legs

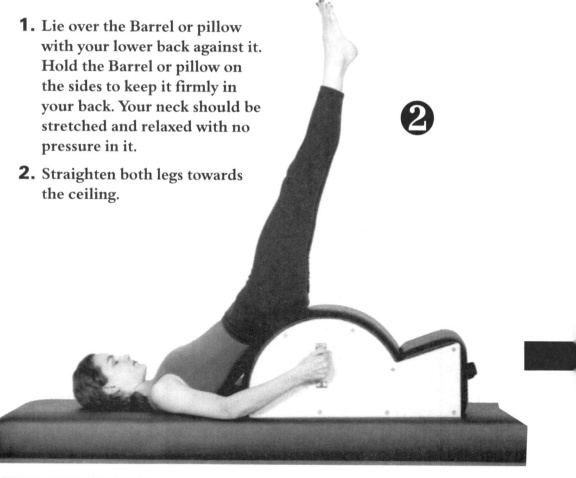

1. Lie over the Barrel or pillow with your lower back against it. Hold the Barrel or pillow on the sides to keep it firmly in your back. Your neck should be stretched and relaxed with no pressure in it.

2. Straighten both legs towards the ceiling.

*"The Pilates® Method changes bodies.
It makes them fitter and stronger and more attractive"*

Philip Friedman and Gail Eisen

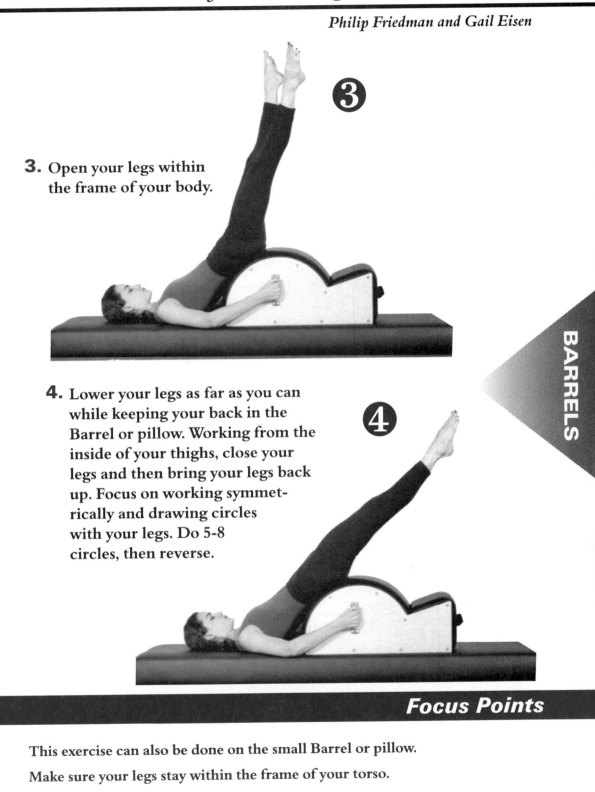

3. Open your legs within
the frame of your body.

4. Lower your legs as far as you can
while keeping your back in the
Barrel or pillow. Working from the
inside of your thighs, close your
legs and then bring your legs back
up. Focus on working symmetrically and drawing circles
with your legs. Do 5-8
circles, then reverse.

BARRELS

Focus Points

This exercise can also be done on the small Barrel or pillow.

Make sure your legs stay within the frame of your torso.

Don't arch your lower back.

Maintain navel to spine at all times.

Exercise 39
Walking

Coordinate legs while working the Powerhouse

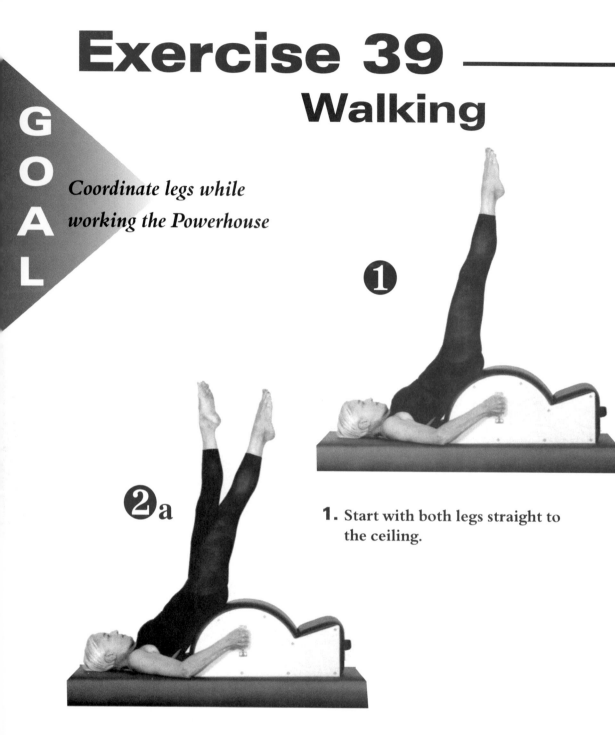

1. Start with both legs straight to the ceiling.

2a., 2b., 2c. Walk your legs down to the mat. Maintain even steps and go only as far down as you can control your back on the Barrel or pillow. With the same control, walk your legs back up. Repeat 3-5 sets.

"The single most effective exercise technique I have ever known."

Actress Stefanie Powers

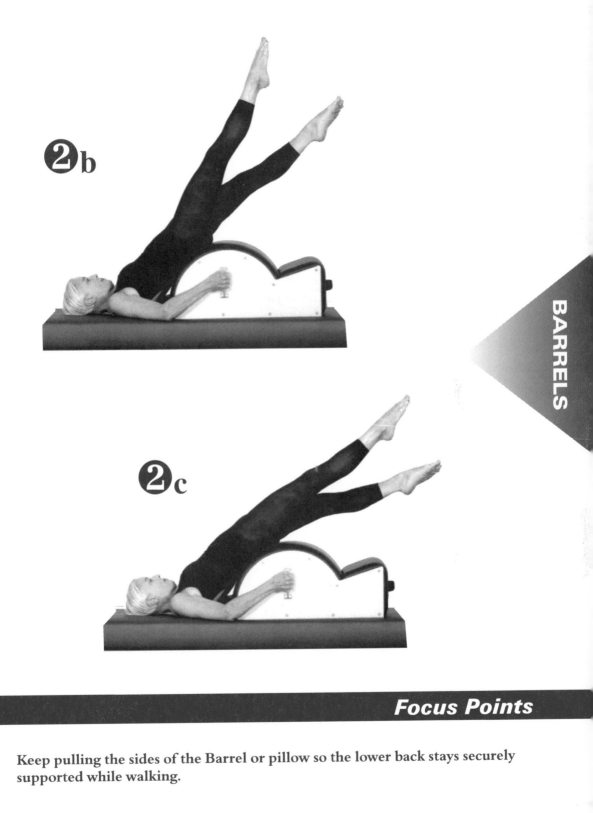

②b

②c

Focus Points

Keep pulling the sides of the Barrel or pillow so the lower back stays securely supported while walking.

Exercise 40
Bicycle

To lengthen your thigh and calf muscles and support your back

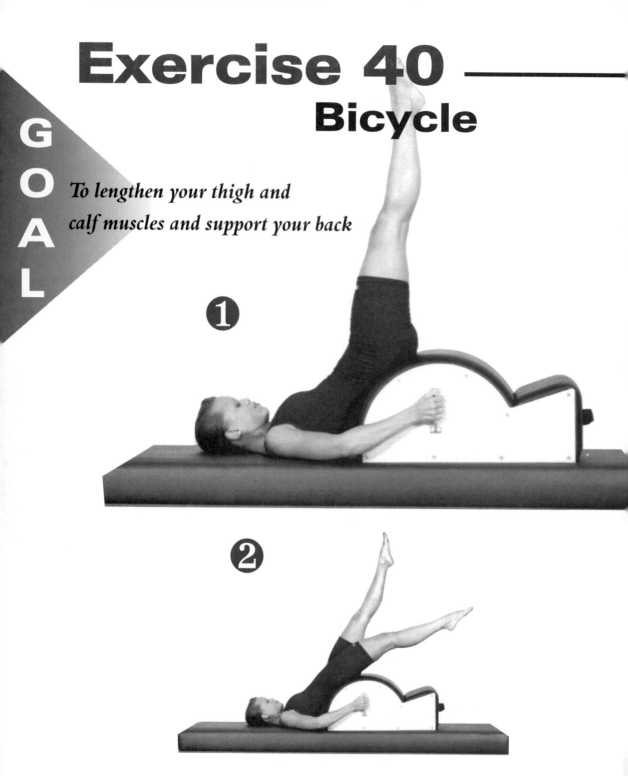

①

②

1. Begin in the same position as in Exercise 39.

2. Reach up towards the ceiling with one leg and down with the other.

The Pilates® Method

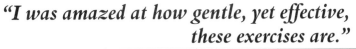

"I was amazed at how gentle, yet effective, these exercises are."

Tennis star Pat Cash

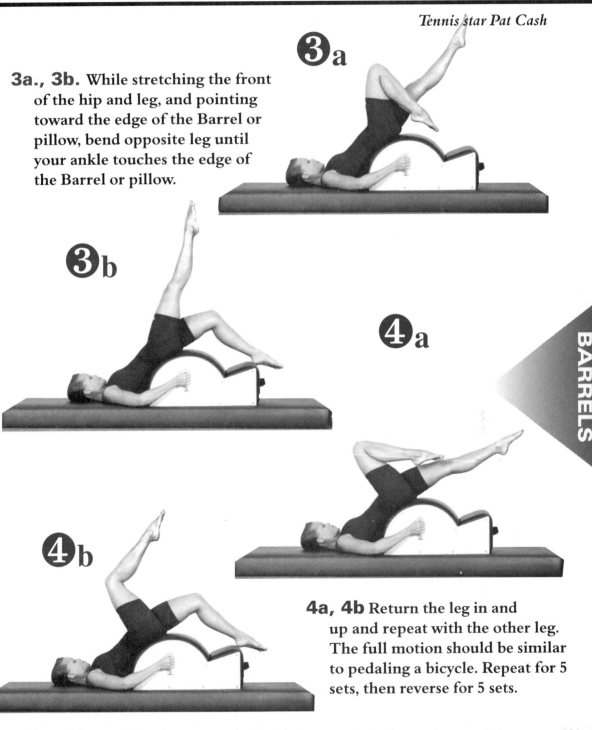

3a., **3b.** While stretching the front of the hip and leg, and pointing toward the edge of the Barrel or pillow, bend opposite leg until your ankle touches the edge of the Barrel or pillow.

❸a

❸b

❹a

❹b

4a, 4b Return the leg in and up and repeat with the other leg. The full motion should be similar to pedaling a bicycle. Repeat for 5 sets, then reverse for 5 sets.

Focus Points

Keep your back on the Barrel or pillow with your belly pulled in.

Focus on the downward leg. Try each time to touch the edge of the Barrel or pillow while increasing your stretch.

Exercise 41
Scissors

G
O
A
L

To slim down bulky thighs and buttocks

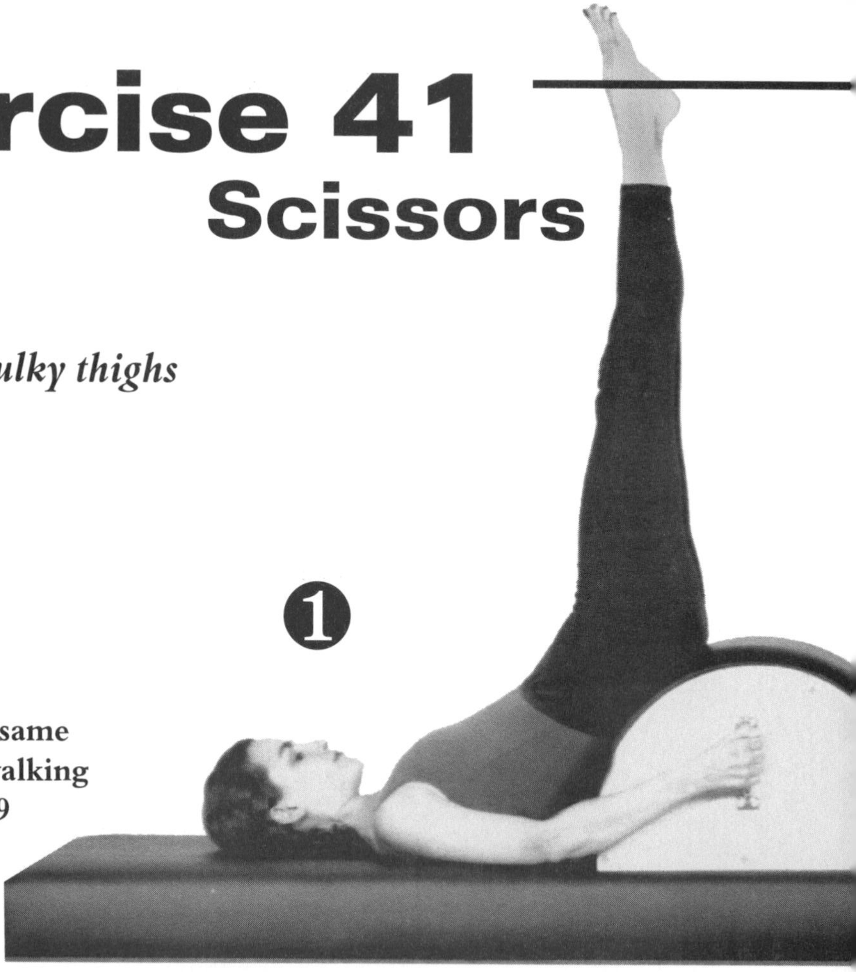

①

1. Begin in the same
position as walking
in Exercise 39

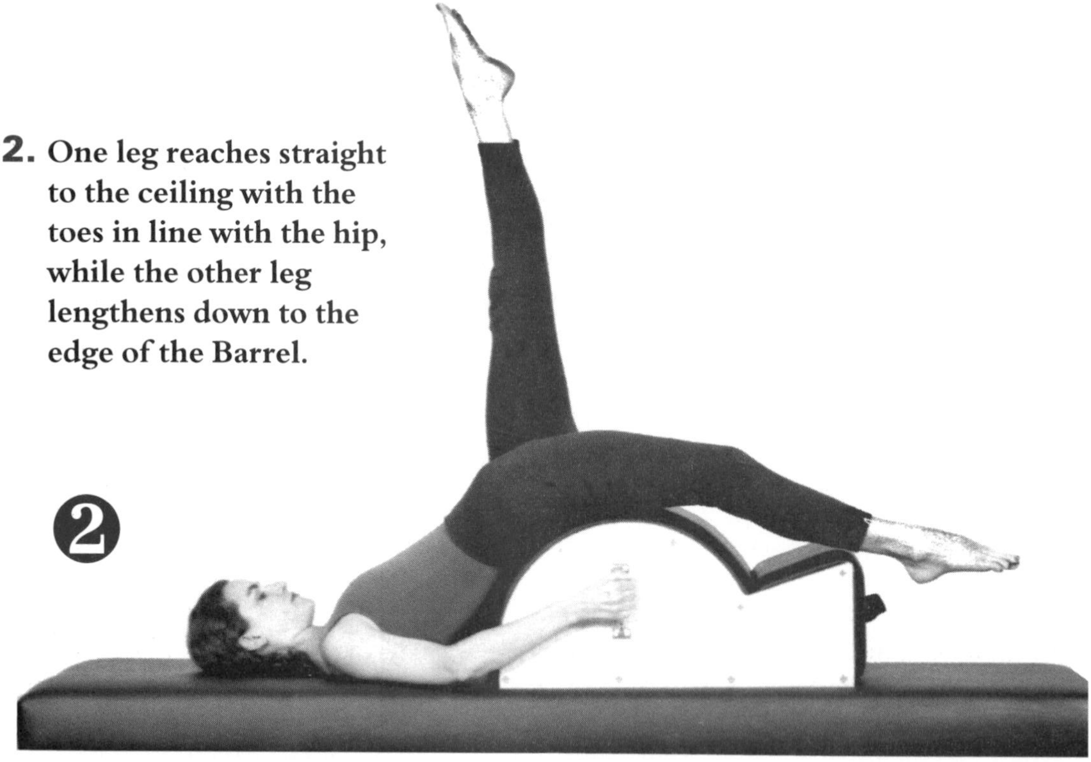

2. One leg reaches straight
to the ceiling with the
toes in line with the hip,
while the other leg
lengthens down to the
edge of the Barrel.

②

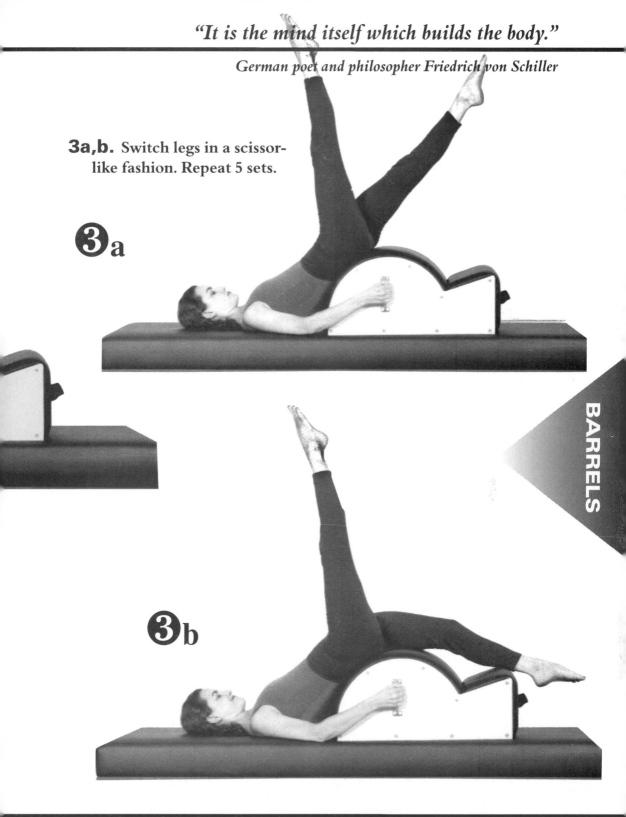

"It is the mind itself which builds the body."

German poet and philosopher Friedrich von Schiller

3a,b. Switch legs in a scissor-like fashion. Repeat 5 sets.

❸a

❸b

Focus Points

Focus on the leg reaching down, opening the hip. Do not let the upward leg fall back over your head.

Exercise 42
Beats

To strengthen your inner and outer thighs and support your back

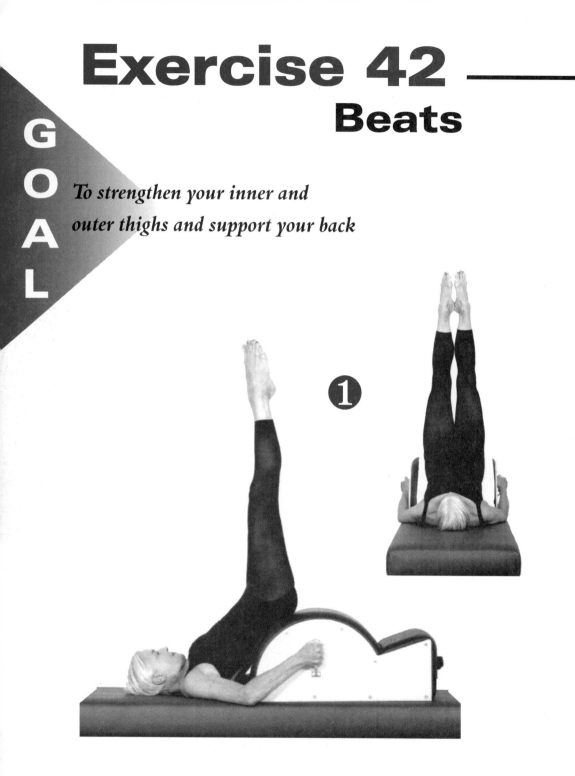

1. Begin in the same position as Walking as in Exercise 39.

"What is balance of body and mind? It is the conscious control of all muscular movements of the body."

Joseph H. Pilates, Your Health, 1934

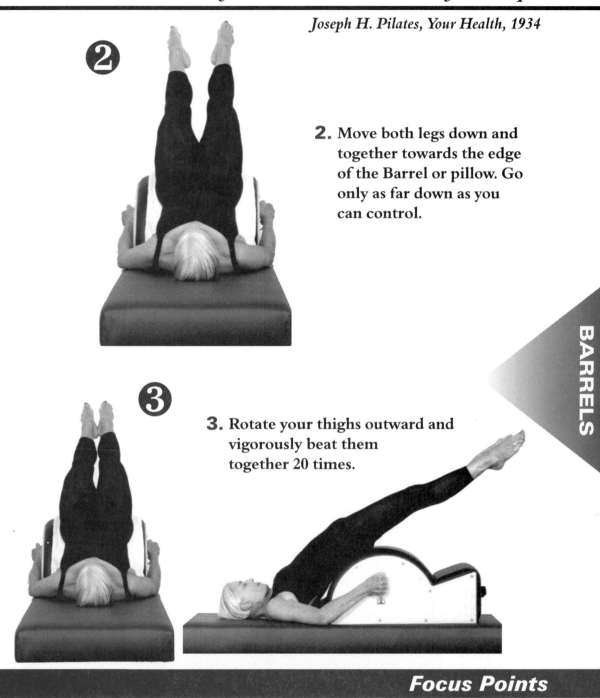

2. Move both legs down and together towards the edge of the Barrel or pillow. Go only as far down as you can control.

3. Rotate your thighs outward and vigorously beat them together 20 times.

BARRELS

Focus Points

If you experience pain or strain in the lower back, your legs are going to far down.

Make certain your legs stay level and that your body does not rotate right or left.

Exercise 43
Rolling In and Out

Massage your lower back after
previous exercises, and for toning fleshy hips

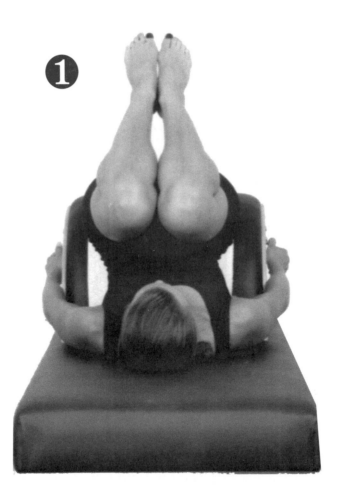

1. Begin in the same position as Walking in
   Exercise 39. Bend your knees into your chest.

"After discovering Pilates, I'm breathing properly, I'm stronger, I'm focused, and I'm relaxed. And I'm skiing better than ever."

Pro ski racer Jessie McAleer

2. With your knees together, roll the lower half of your body from right to left.

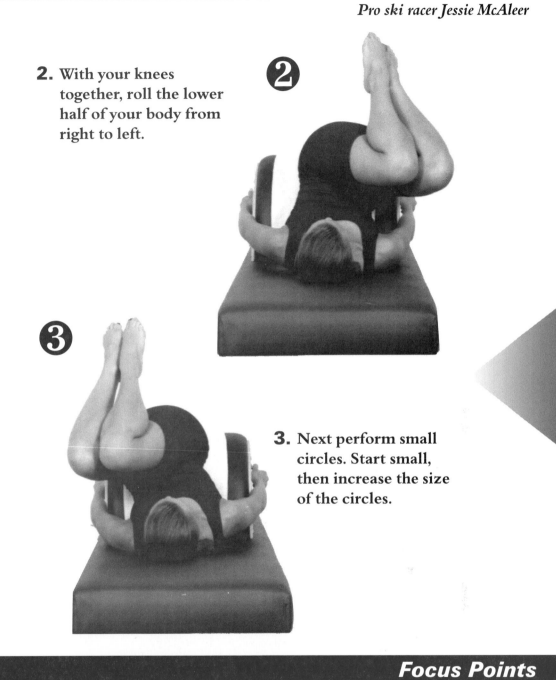

3. Next perform small circles. Start small, then increase the size of the circles.

Focus Points

To finish the Leg Series, carefully push the Barrel away until you lie flat on your back with the knees over the Barrel. Rest. Breathe naturally.

Part 6
The Pilates® Performer™

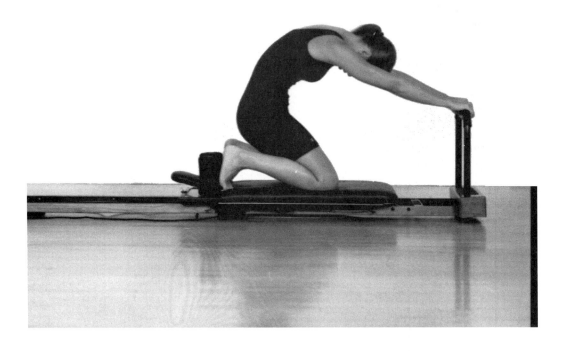

*The Pilates® Performer™ is the home
version of the Universal Reformer which
is found in the Pilates Studios®. The
Performer provides a wide range of
exercises, from simple to intermediate,
in order to develop the Powerhouse.
It contains straps, springs, and a box
for activities devoted to improving most
muscles and joints. When you master the
Performer you exercise in constant, fluid
movement with the minimum of effort.*

Objectives:

Alignment of the body

Circulation of the blood

Endurance

Expanding the breath

Anchoring the spine

Slendering the thighs and buttocks

Opening out the lower back

Working the internal organs

Lengthening the lower back

*Strengthen the Powerhouse, hips,
        legs and lower abdominals*

Articulate the vertibrae

Lengthen the torso

Stretch the spine and back of the leg

Balance and alignment control

Working the waist and strengthening the sides

Opening the shoulders

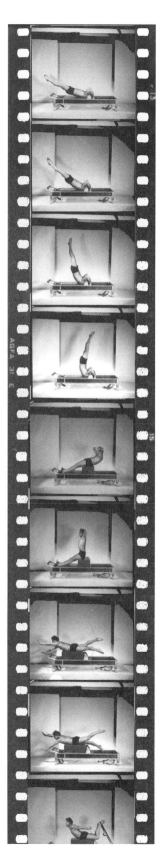

Exercise 44a
Footwork 1

Centering, concentrating and aligning the body

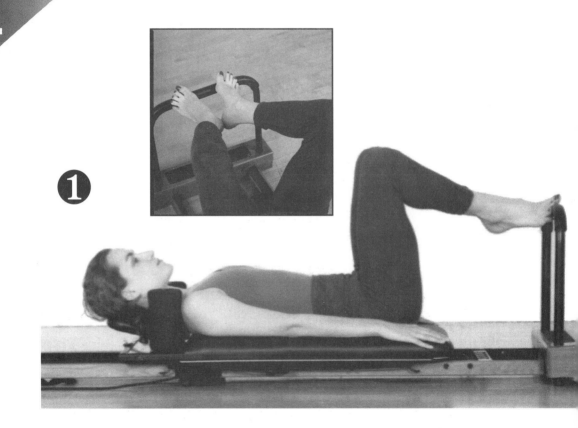

①

Spring Setting: 4 springs (3 springs for those under 110 pounds)

1. Lie on your back with your knees up and bring your stomach muscles in. Center yourself correctly. Place your toes on the bar. Keep your toes apart and your heels together and lifted. Your knees should be shoulder width apart.

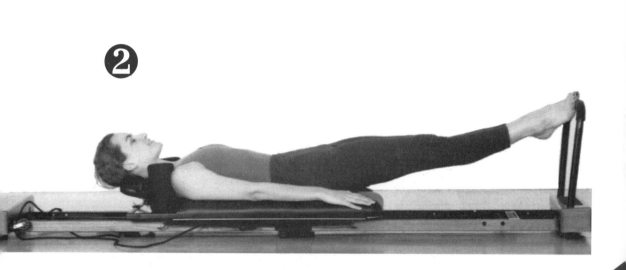

2. In this position, initiate from the Powerhouse and push the carriage fully out, straightening the legs. Using your Powerhouse, return the carriage to the starting position. With control, push and pull with a smooth continuous motion, working the springs. Do 10 repetitions, then work your arches.

See next page for steps 3 through 5

PERFORMER

Focus Points

This is the most important exercise in the Performer workout as it aligns and strengthens your body.

Use pads to protect your feet.

Make sure the Powerhouse is always initiating the movement of the carriage. Abdominal and gluteal muscles work to stabilize you while in action.

If you are knock-kneed, work with your feet hip width apart. Your back should stay flat and your shoulders and neck relaxed. Shoulder pads can be used for comfort.

Exercise 44b
Footwork 2

*Centering, concentrating
and aligning the body*

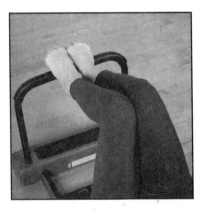

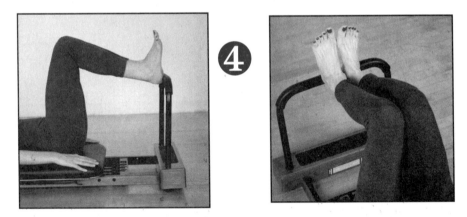

3. For your arches, repeat the exercise with your arches on the bar like a bird on a perch. Keep your feet and knees together while working. Do 10 repetitions.

4. Repeat the exercise with your heels on the bar. Your knees and feet remain firmly together while pushing out and in. As you come in, pull your toes towards your knees. Do 10 repetitions, then work your tendons.

⑤

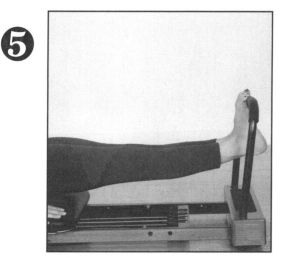

PERFORMER

5. Place your toes back on the bar slightly apart with heels together. Push the carriage out and stay there as you lower your heels for 3 counts and lift for 3 counts. Work the upper part of your legs to avoid working with hyper-extended knees.

Focus Points

See Focus Points on previous exercise.

Exercise 45
The Hundred

Expand the breath, blood circulation and endurance

①

Spring Setting: 4 springs

1. Place the footbar down and grab hold of the strap handles behind you.

2. Lift your head and bring your towards your chest. The weight of your head should be leaning into the center of your body. Lift your legs to a 90 degree angle with toes pointing toward the ceiling. Straighten your arms, pulling the straps down to your sides about 6 to 8 inches above your thighs.

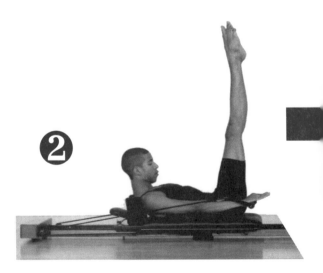

②

The Pilates® Method

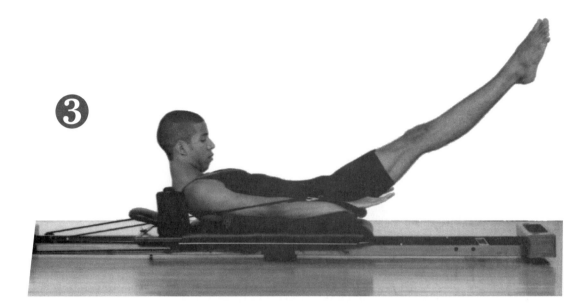

3. Straighten your legs out at an angle. Work with long, soft legs. Pump your arms up and down for 10 deep breaths. Inhale through the nose for 5 counts and exhale through the nose for 5 counts. Your arms should be energized, pumping vigorously to get the blood circulating.

PERFORMER

Focus Points

If you have already done the Hundred in your Mat work (see Exercise 1) you may omit this exercise.

In Step 3 only lower your legs as low as you can control from the Powerhouse. The lower back must remain flat and not arched.

Begin with only 20 movements, then gradually increase until the maximum of 100 is reached.

In this exercise, your legs should be at eye level. If you are not able to do this without arching your back, raise your legs to an angle where you can keep your back flat.

Exercise 46
Coordination

GOAL

Coordination and exercising the lungs

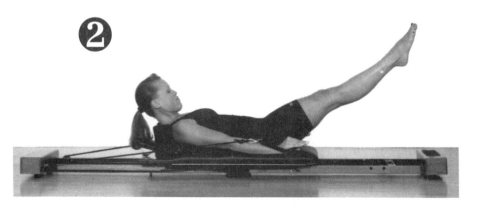

❶

Spring Setting: 4 springs

1. Lift your chin into your chest and bend your knees into your body. Bend your elbows into your sides at a 90 degree angle.

2. From this position, inhale as you straighten your arms and legs. Your elbows and forearms should touch the mat.

❷

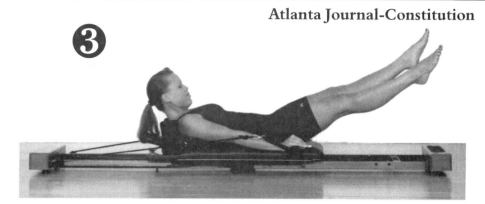

3. While holding your breath, smoothly open and close your legs. Open your legs no wider than the frame.

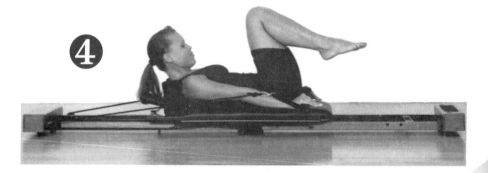

4. Exhale as you bend your knees back towards your chest.

5. Continue to exhale, fully emptying your lungs, while bending your arms back to the starting position. Repeat a maximum of 5 times.

PERFORMER

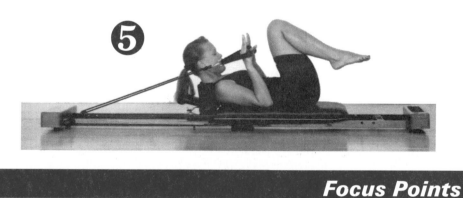

Focus Points

Bring your legs as low as you can while maintaining a flat back.

Your wrists should remain straight while pulling the straps.

Exercise 47
Long Stretch

Forming a long Powerhouse

①

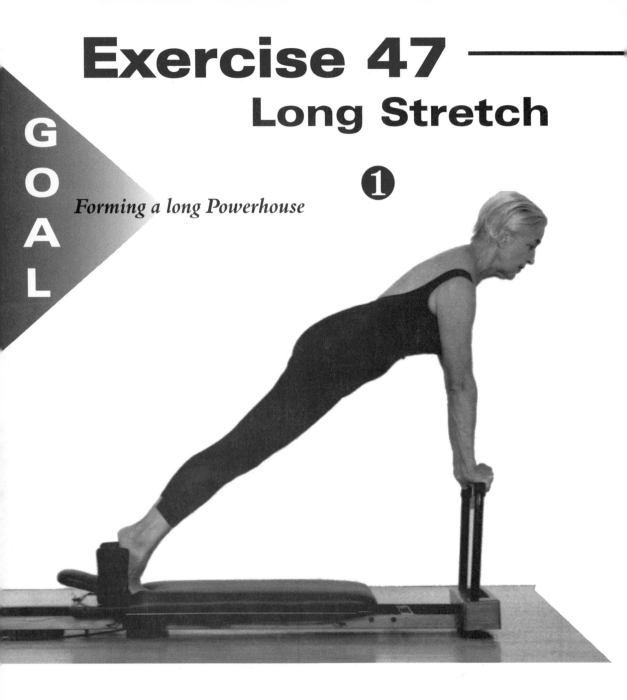

Spring Setting: 2 springs

1. Get on the Performer placing one hand on the foot bar first, then one foot on the center-front of the head-piece. Then place your other hand and foot as shown. With your feet in between the shoulder blocks, heels over toes and hands on the footbar, lengthen yourself into a push up position.

The Pilates® Method

2. Keeping your body in a straight line, push the carriage out, working the buttocks, hips and abdominals. Inhale as you push out.

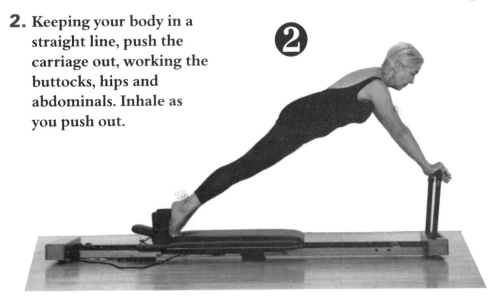

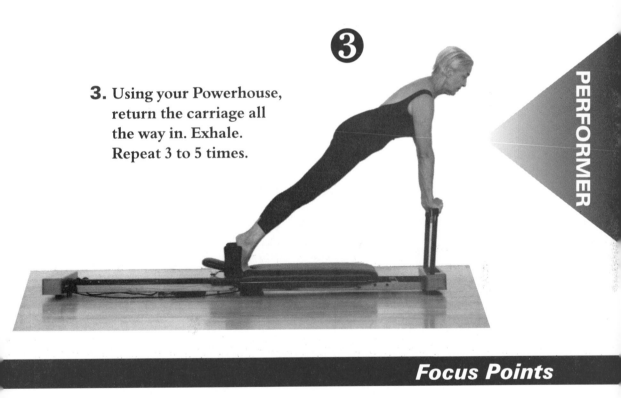

3. Using your Powerhouse, return the carriage all the way in. Exhale. Repeat 3 to 5 times.

PERFORMER

Focus Points

CAUTION: Do not pull on the bar, only push! You can have a partner or trainer stand next to the Performer and hold the bar in place with his or her foot just in case.

In this exercise, it is not about how far you push the carriage out as much as it is using your Powerhouse to bring the carriage out and in.

Exercise 48
Down Stretch

Working the lungs and exhaling

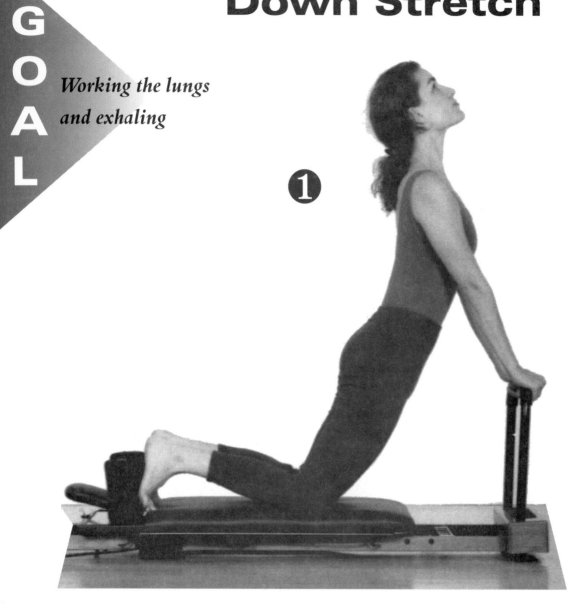

①

Spring Setting: 2 springs

1. Kneel down. Place your feet flexed in front of the shoulder blocks. Go into an upper back bend. Stay lifted in your lower back and abdominal wall.

2

2. Inhale as you push the carriage back. Maintain this lifted position.

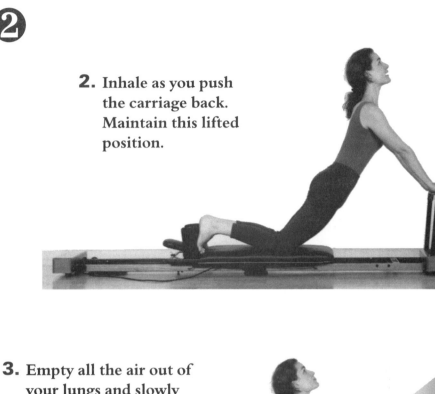

3

3. Empty all the air out of your lungs and slowly bring the carriage in. Increase your lift and back bend when the carriage is in. Repeat a maximum of 3 times.

PERFORMER

Focus Points

Make sure your back stays supported while in this arched position by using your abdomen. Do not go out too far. The dynamics of the exercise are in and up.

Exercise 49
Up Stretch

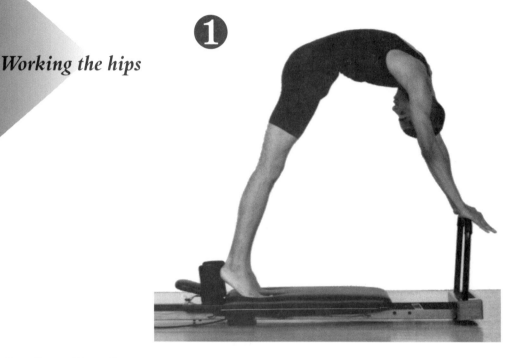

Spring Settings: 2 springs

1. Rise up on the balls of your feet and fold your body in half. Point your nose your knees. Lift in your ribs and scoop the abdominals in and up.

2. Using your hips and Powerhouse, push the carriage out as you inhale. Working your buttocks, curl your tailbone under and down so your body is once again in a straight line. Relax your head to your chest.

The Pilates® Method

"We should recognize the mental functions of the mind and the physical limitations of the body so that complete coordination between them may be achieved."

Joseph H. Pilates, Your Health

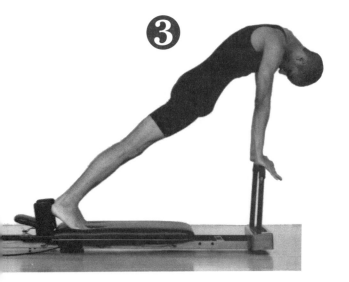

3. Exhaling, bring the carriage all the way in, maintaining your long line.

4. Keep the carriage in, then fold yourself in half, pointing the crown of your head down. Do 3-4 repetitions.

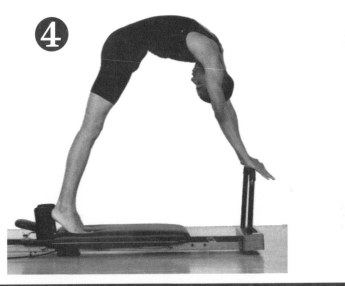

PERFORMER

Focus Points

Make sure your body stays in one straight line, firmly supported by your hips, buttocks and abdominals. A partner or trainer can assist you by placing one hand on your back and the other on your abdomen for support until you get the feeling of the exercise.

The focus of the exercise is on the incoming motion. Beware of pushing out too far and losing lower back support.

Exercise 50

Elephant

Isolate the abdomen, strengthen the hips and stretch the calves and hamstrings

①

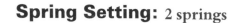

Spring Setting: 2 springs

1. Place your heels down on the mat in front of the shoulder blocks. Lift your toes. Bring your stomach muscles in and drop your head and shoulders. Brace your upper body against the bar.

The Pilates® Method

"Joe Pilates didn't believe in what he called 'unnatural exercise' – forcing the body into strained postures or repeating the same motions to the point of exhaustion."

Philip Friedman and Gail Eisen

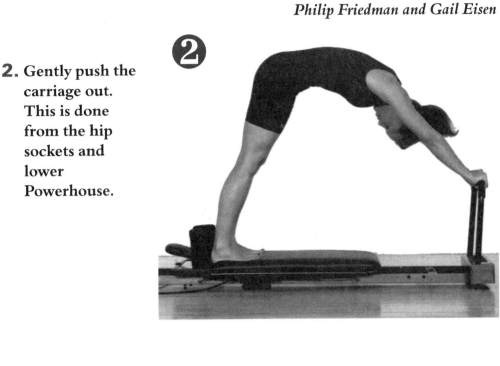

2. Gently push the carriage out. This is done from the hip sockets and lower Powerhouse.

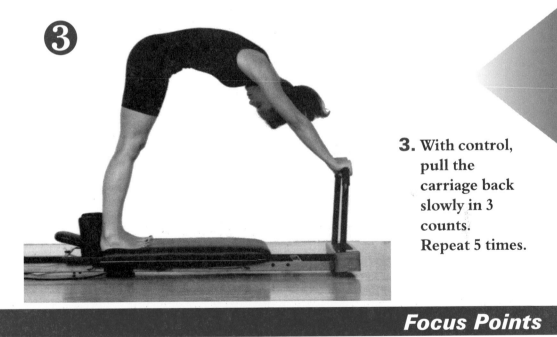

PERFORMER

3. With control, pull the carriage back slowly in 3 counts. Repeat 5 times.

Focus Points

Make sure you push your hips out using your lower abdominal muscles.
Keep your rib cage and diaphragm lifted into your back without movement.

It is important you slow down the rhythm on the return carriage movement.
Dig your heels into the Mat to work on your calves.

Exercise 51
Stomach Massage: Round

"C-Curve," open out the lower back and work the internal organs

①

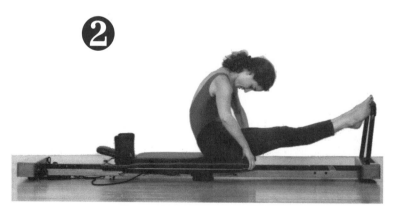

Spring Setting: 3 springs

1. Sit on the Performer facing forward with your tailbone curved under. Place your toes on the footbar toes apart heels together. Place your hands on the edge of the mat with your elbows out. Bring your shoulders over your hips and relax your head forward.

②

The Pilates® Method

> *"The Pilates method can be used by everyone, regardless of age or physical limitations."*
>
> *Aliesa George-Jefferies, owner Flinthills Physical Conditioning, Wichita, Kansas*

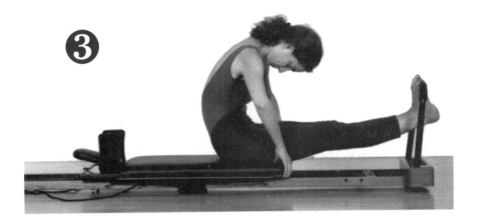

2. Maintaining this position, use your Powerhouse to straighten your legs. Bring your stomach muscles in to initiate five repetitions. Keep your heels together.

3. Lower and lift your heels.

4. Return to starting position.

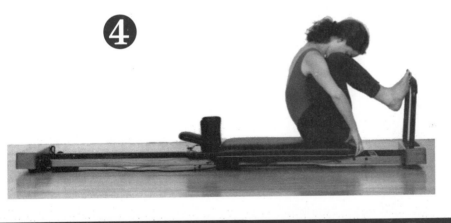

Focus Points

Use a pad to protect your toes.

Make sure your stomach gets its massage! Do not push out with the legs.

At all times your sit bones should remain under and the lower back should remain in a "C-curve." Your shoulders, neck and head should be relaxed.

Keep your elbows out to get a stretch across the upper back and to firm the underarm muscles.

Exercise 52

Stomach Massage: Hands Back

Lengthen the lower back and open the upper back

1

Spring Setting: 2 springs

1. Bring your arms behind you and brace your hands against the shoulder blocks. Place balls of feet on the bar as shown. Hand position can vary depending on the individual. While your tailbone remains underneath, lift your upper back and open your chest.

"I don't have some of the bulges. It's like liposuction."

Philadelphia business executive Susan Goldberg

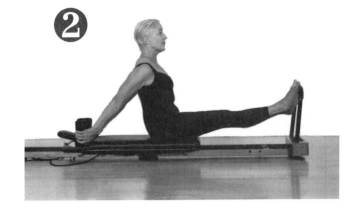

2. From your center, push the carriage out.

3. Lower and lift your heels, maintaining a correct alignment in your legs to prevent your knees from rolling in.

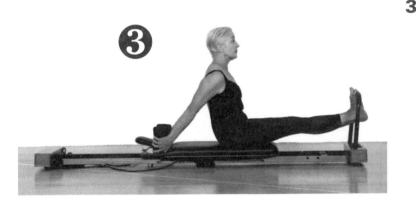

PERFORMER

4. Return to the starting position. Repeat 10 times.

Focus Points

Use pads to protect your feet.

Note: Hold onto your "C-curve." Open only the upper back to expand the lungs. Make sure your back is as high and straight as possible.

Do not allow your elbows to hyperextend.

Inhale as the carriage moves out and the heels lower. Exhale while returning.

Exercise 53
Stomach Massage: Reach-Up

Open the lower back and lift the Powerhouse

①

Spring Setting:
2 springs

1. Place your heels together and toes apart on the bar and straighten your back as shown. Reach forward with your arms in a high diagonal.

The Pilates® Method

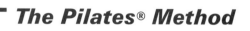

"Each time you do the movements, you come away feeling stimulated and renewed."

Philip Friedman and Gail Eisen

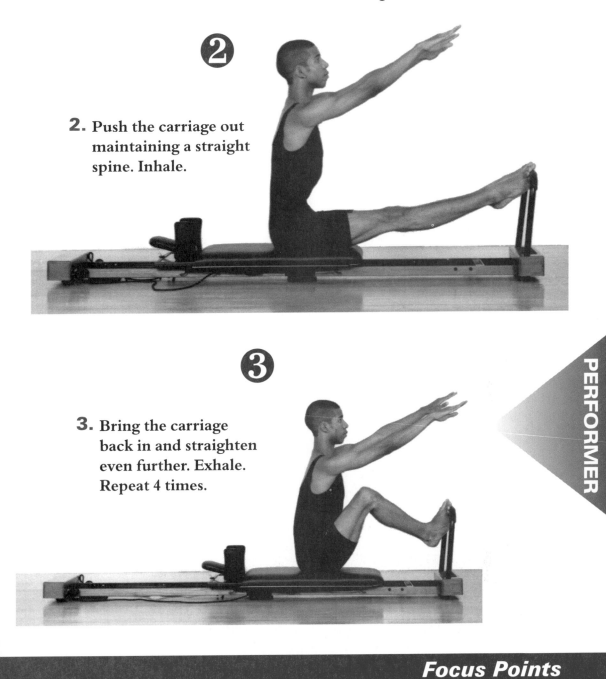

2. Push the carriage out maintaining a straight spine. Inhale.

3. Bring the carriage back in and straighten even further. Exhale. Repeat 4 times.

PERFORMER

Focus Points

Make sure you lift your back from the base of your spine and not from the shoulders or arms. Engage the Powerhouse.

For individuals with very stiff backs, a partner or trainer can assist with this exercise by gently pulling your back forward and upward or by pushing upward in your lower back.

149

*Empty your lungs
and correct your posture*

①

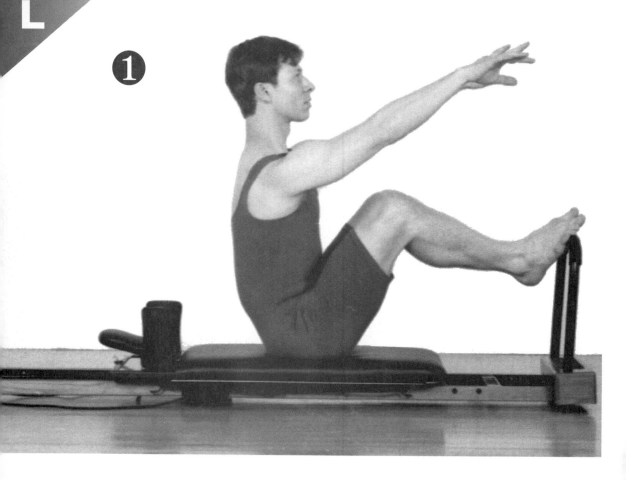

Spring Setting: 2 springs

1. Start in the Reach-Up forward position.
(See Exercise 53.)

2. As you push the carriage out, twist your torso. Open your shoulder and chest and reach your right arm to the right, looking behind you. Your shoulder should stay over your hip.

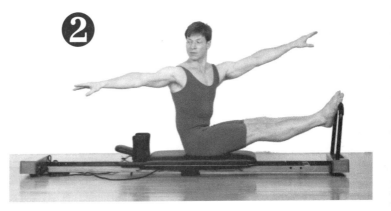

3. Return the carriage in and reach up when you are back center.

PERFORMER

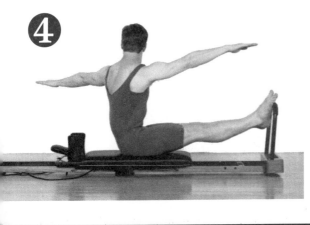

4. Repeat to the left. Inhale as you twist and exhale as you reach forward. Repeat 3 times on each side.

Focus Points

Make sure you keep your spine straight as you twist.

The twist happens in the waist. Your pelvis should stay centered. Keep your heels together as you twist.

Exercise 55
Knee Stretch: Round

Work the upper back, Powerhouse and chest

①

Spring Setting: 2 springs

1. Starting from the Round position (see Exercise 51), arch your upper back. Lift your chest and pelvis. Keep your tailbone towards your heels.

> *"Imagine the immediate good resulting if the energies that are now so wastefully expended were directed into the road to normal health!"*
>
> *Joseph H. Pilates*

2. Push the carriage out.

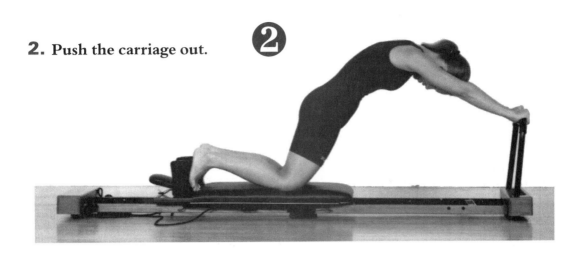

3. With an accent, pull the carriage back in. Repeat 6-8 times.

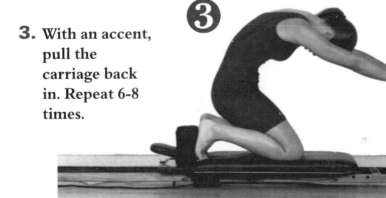

PERFORMER

Focus Points

The same principles apply here as to the Round (Exercise 51).

CAUTION: People with a weak lower back should proceed cautiously with this exercise. Gradually work into this arched position.

Exercise 56
Knee Stretch Arched

*Arch the upper back,
open the chest and
counter massage*

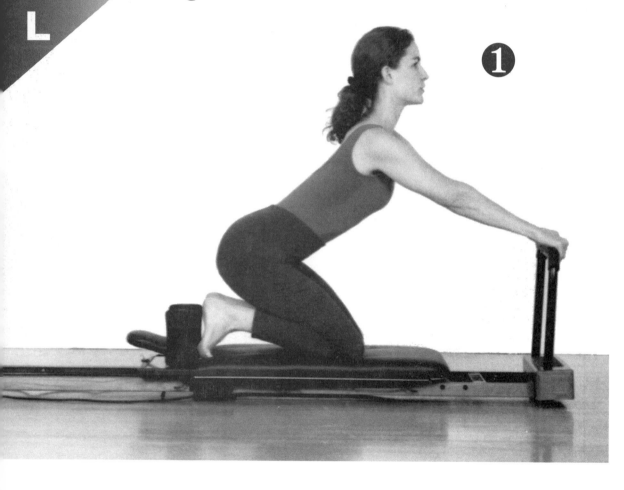

①

Spring Setting: 2 springs

1. Starting from the round position, arch the upper back,
lifting the chest and the pelvis.

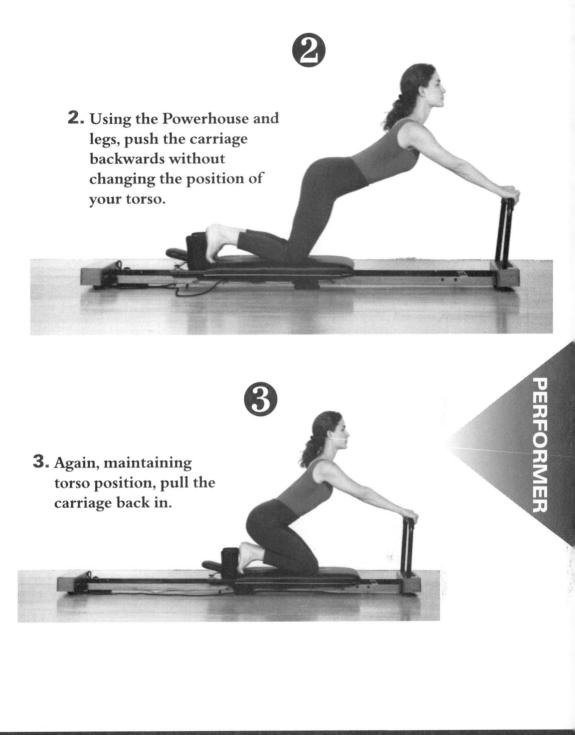

2. Using the Powerhouse and legs, push the carriage backwards without changing the position of your torso.

3. Again, maintaining torso position, pull the carriage back in.

PERFORMER

Focus Points

CAUTION: People with a weak lower back should proceed cautiously with this exercise. Work into this arched position gradually.

Exercise 57
Knee Stretch: Knees Off

Strengthening the legs and Powerhouse

①

Spring Setting: 2 springs

1. Return to the C-Curve position (see Exercise 51, Page 144). Lift your knees off the mat with your tailbone curled under and your head relaxed and down, chin pointing to chest. Lift your knees to ankle height. Bring your body weight further forward.

"I'm totally addicted. I know that my own flexibility and strength have increased dramatically since starting Pilates."

Betsy Frampton, Washington, D.C. businesswoman

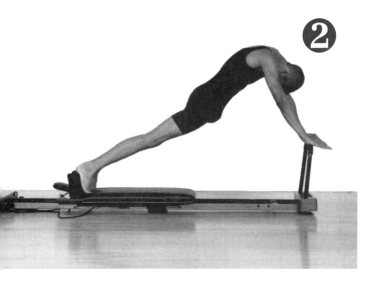

2. Straighten your knees all the way, maintaining a strong Powerhouse.

3. Bend your knees to pull the carriage in with an accent on the "in" movement. Repeat 8-10 times.

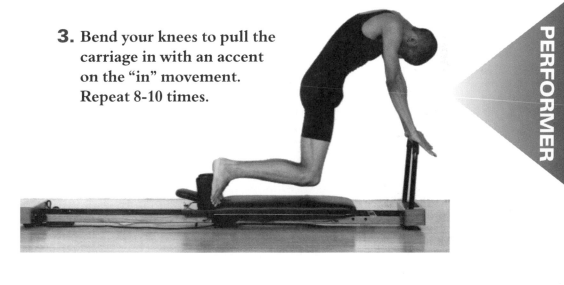

PERFORMER

Focus Points

NOTE: For beginners, your knees might not straighten all the way. Introduce this gradually.

If you have tender knees or have trouble finding this position with your body, do this variation: Start by standing up on the carriage. Lift your heels up against the shoulder blocks as if you were going to do the Up Stretch (see Exercise 49). From this position, scoop the tailbone under, bending and lowering your knees until they are at ankle height.

Exercise 58

Running

*Cool down,
return to your center*

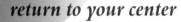

①

②

1. Lie on your back with your toes placed on the footbar. Your legs should be parallel. Centering the spine, bring your stomach muscles in.

2. Push the carriage out.

3. Lower one heel and bend the opposite knee, lifting your ankle to work the arch. Keep your knees pointed straight up. Repeat 20 times.

4. Switch legs. Repeat 20 times.

The Pilates® Method

"People comment on how good you look; your clothes fit differently. You don't have those daytime energy dips."

Philip Friedman and Gail Eisen

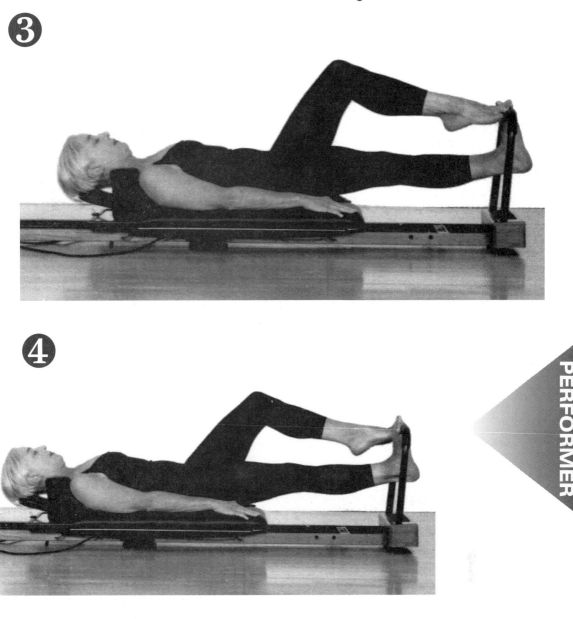

③

④

PERFORMER

Focus Points

Make sure your knees stay properly aligned, that is always pointed straight up. If necessary, open your toes and keep your heels together to do this.

The gluteal and abdominal muscles should be working to keep your hips from swaying.

The rhythm of this exercise is "springy." Work the ankle and arch evenly.

Exercise 59

Long Box: Pulling Straps

Opening the lungs and chest, strengthen shoulders and upper back

1

Spring Settings: 1 Spring

1. Facing the back of the Performer, lie on your stomach on the box as shown. Your shoulders should be flush with the back edge of the box. With outstretched arms hold high up on the straps and bring them towards the outside of the frame.

2. Inhaling, pull the straps downward close to the body and along the frame. Continue pulling them back as you lift and open the chest. Hold this position for 3 counts.

3. With control, lower your body back to the box while exhaling. Continue with Exercise 60.

> *"After trying Pilates for myself I began to encourage many of my patients to take it up, with astonishing results."*
>
> Osteopath Piers Chandler

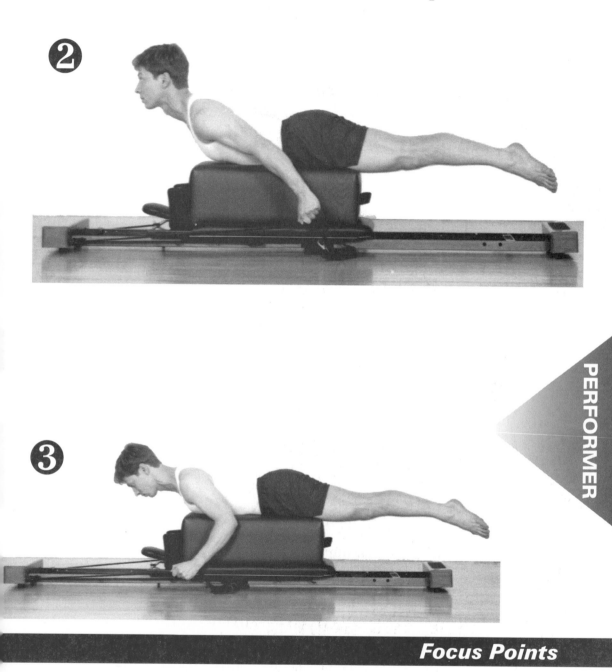

PERFORMER

Focus Points

Bring shoulder blades together in the back.

Do not over-arch the neck.

Pull belly in and squeeze the buttocks.

(The box is available from the Pilates Studio®. See Page 207.)

Exercise 60
Long Box: Pulling Straps, T-Shape

Work the chest, upper body and shoulders

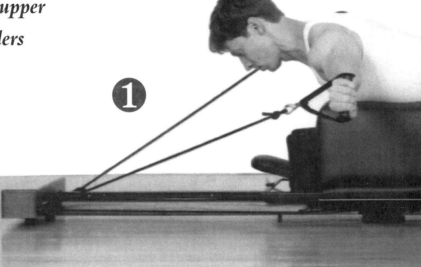

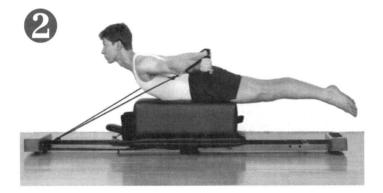

1. Upon completing Exercise 59, slide your hands down to the end of the straps. Open your arms to the sides, lifting them to shoulder height.

2. Keep your arms at shoulder height and pull them back, lifting and opening the chest.

3. Exhaling, lower down the box. Do 3 repetitions.

The Pilates® Method

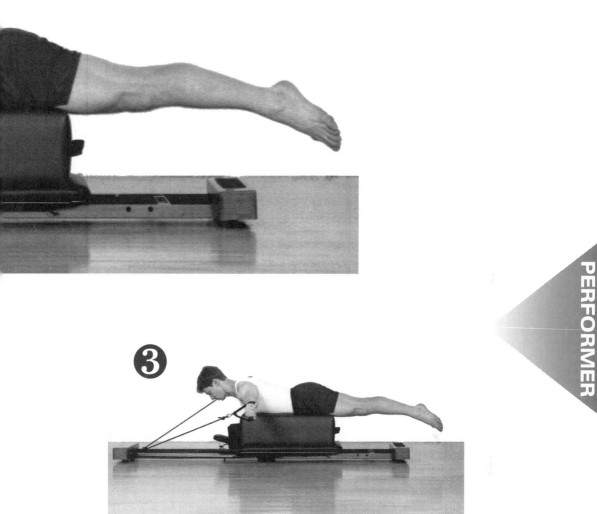

PERFORMER

Focus Points

Make sure you work the upper back and not the neck only. Keep the neck long and straight.

Keep your legs low and in the Pilates stance. Work the upper back, not the lower back.

Part 7
Chair Exercises

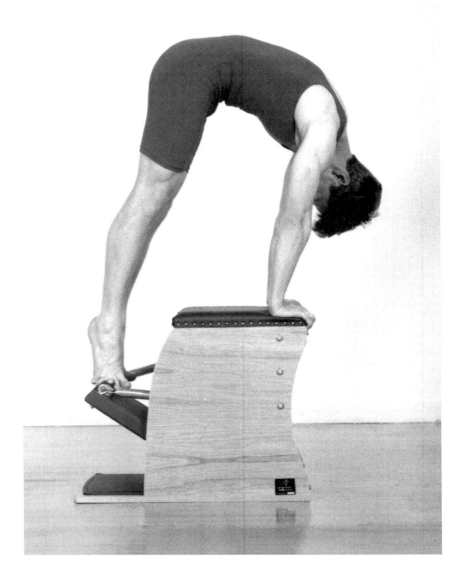

The Pilates® Method

The Chair was developed by Joseph H. Pilates to stretch and strengthen muscle groups which are not easily reached by more traditional techniques and equipment. It provides exercises that offer great balance and control of the body. It forms the basis of an entire range of advanced Pilates exercises.

Objectives:

Ultimate balance and control

Stretch the spine

Strengthen the Powerhouse

Stretch the hamstrings

Strengthen the legs and feet

Strengthen the hamstrings,
*   calves and Achilles tendons*

Strengthen the glutes and arms

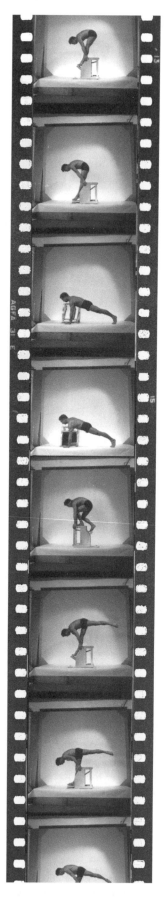

Exercise 61
Push Down

To stretch your hamstrings and strengthen your Powerhouse

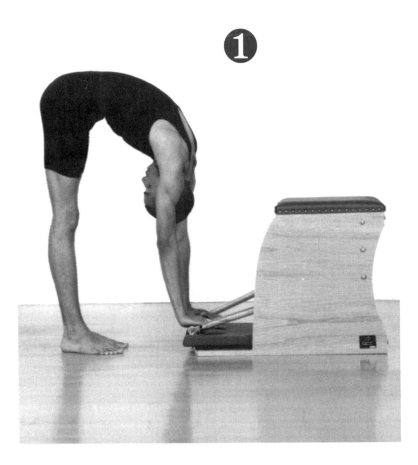

①

1. Place 1 spring in the middle or 2 springs on the bottom. Stand facing the chair, keeping your hips over your heels. Place your hands on the pedal. Press the pedal straight down.

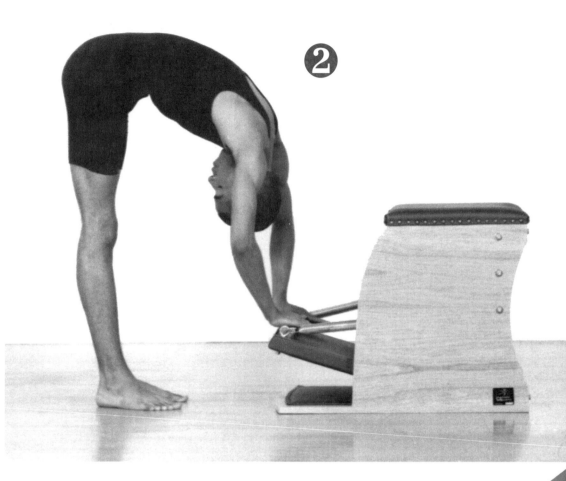

2. Lift the pedal by bending the elbows only. Repeat 3 times. After the third repetition press the pedal down once more. With straight arms, bring the pedal back up using your Powerhouse. Repeat for 3 sets.

THE CHAIR

Focus Points

Make sure you are standing bent or folded over with your hips directly over your heels. Maintain this position throughout the exercise.

Keep the lift small at first to find your Powerhouse. When you know how to initiate from the Powerhouse add the arm movement.

Exercise 62
Pull Up

To strengthen your Powerhouse

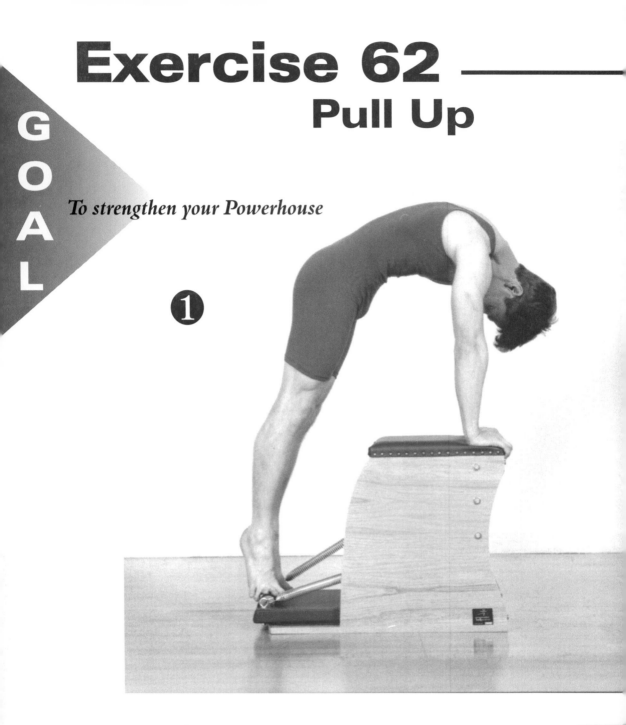

1. Place 1 spring on the top and 1 on the bottom. Facing the chair place both hands on the back edge of the chair and with one foot press the pedal down. Then place the other foot on the pedal, heels together and toes apart.

The Pilates® Method

"The Pilates® Method is a flowing motion outward from a strong center."

Romana Kryzanowska

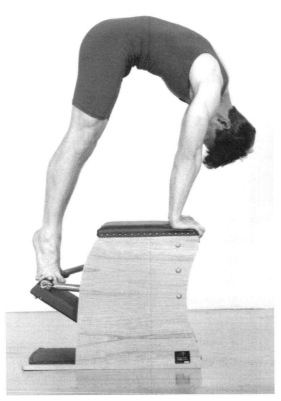

2. Initiating from the Powerhouse, lift the pedal up and hold for 5 counts.

3. With control, lower the pedal and lower the heels for a stretch. Repeat 5 times.

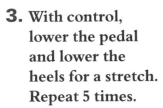

THE CHAIR

Focus Points

It is advisable to first work with a certified instructor on this exercise.

Variation: Rise all the way up, then lower only halfway down and back up. Repeat, then lower the pedal completely down.

Make sure your body remains forward with your legs at a right angle as shown, pelvis over the heels. Maintain this position as the pedal goes up and down.

Inhale on the way up and exhale on the way down.

169

Exercise 63 ———
Arches

To strengthen your legs and feet

①

1. Place the arches of your feet on the pedal like a bird on a perch. Keep your knees and feet together.

The Pilates® Method

"My method develops the body uniformly, corrects wrong postures, restores physical vitality, invigorates the mind and elevates the spirit."

Joseph H. Pilates

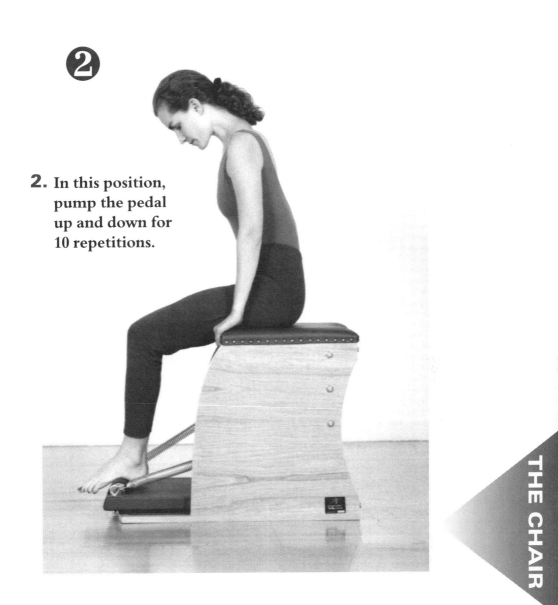

2. In this position, pump the pedal up and down for 10 repetitions.

THE CHAIR

Focus Points

Do not allow your buttocks to lift off the seat of the Chair

CAUTION: Do not do this exercise if you have injured knees.

Exercise 64
Tendon Stretch

GOAL

To strengthen the Powerhouse, hamstrings, calves and Achilles tendon

1

1. Set up the chair the same as for the Pull Up (see Exercise 62). Facing away from the chair, lean on the edge. Put your arches on the pedal and press it down. Place your hands on the front edge of the chair. Bend over forward and bring your nose to your knees.

"After 20 to 30 sessions, you'll look better, feel better, sleep better and experience better sexual enjoyment."

Sean P. Gallagher

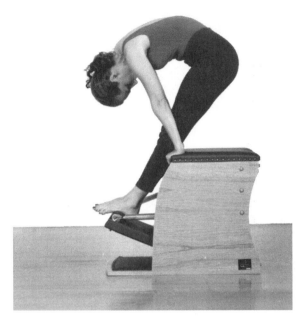

2. Through the Powerhouse, pull the pedal up and hold for 3 counts.

3. With control, release the pedal down. Repeat 3-5 times.

Focus Points

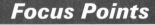

As the pedal rises up the body should remain bent forward. Release your neck and drop your head.

Work the pedal all the way up and all the way down with control but dynamically.

Exercise 65
The Table

To strengthen the glutes, hamstrings, calves and arms

①

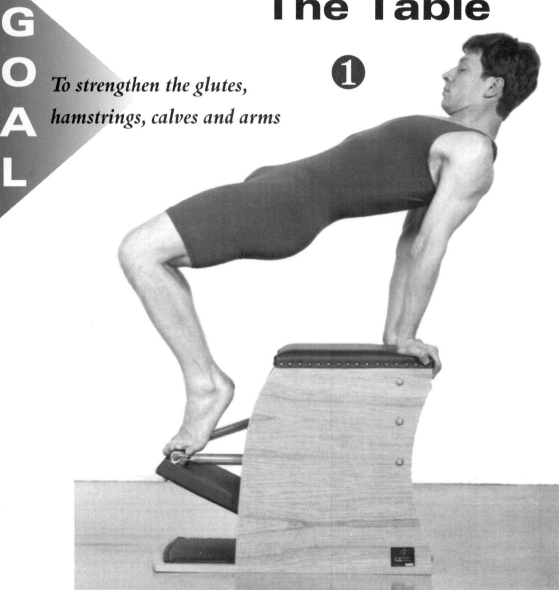

1. Set the chair up the same as for the Pull Up (see Exercise 62). Use a stronger spring setting according to your strength. Sit on the chair and place your hands over the back edge as shown. Place your feet on the pedal with your legs parallel and spread to hip width. Working your buttocks, lift your pelvis up.

"If you spend about 3 hours a week on Pilates, we believe you will attain superb body conditioning and excellent mental well-being."

Sean P. Gallagher and Romana Kryzanowska

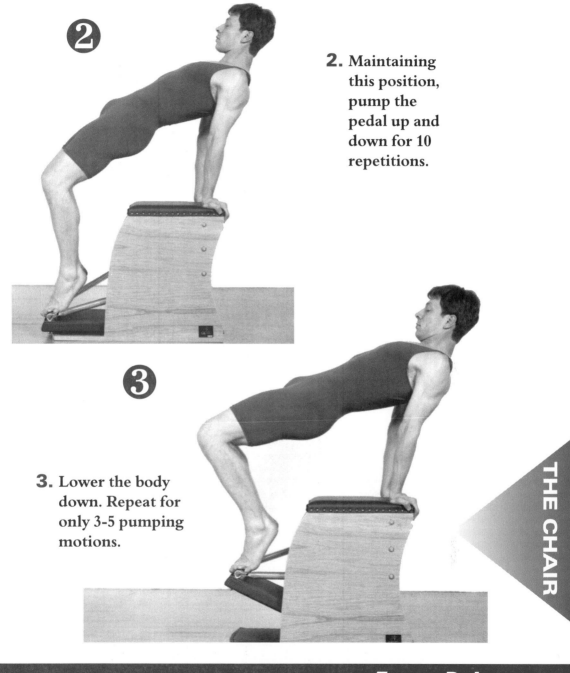

2. Maintaining this position, pump the pedal up and down for 10 repetitions.

3. Lower the body down. Repeat for only 3-5 pumping motions.

THE CHAIR

Focus Points

Variation: The pumping can be done one leg at a time while the other leg is forward and up.

While pumping, make sure your upper body stays still and your pelvis is lifted as high as possible, making your front "flat as a table top."

Exercise 66
Spine Stretch

To maintain the Powerhouse
While stretching the spine

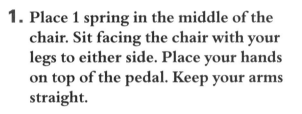

1. Place 1 spring in the middle of the chair. Sit facing the chair with your legs to either side. Place your hands on top of the pedal. Keep your arms straight.

"Pilates tapped my muscle imbalances, highlighting my weak links and how to compensate for them."

Ski Champion Kate McBride

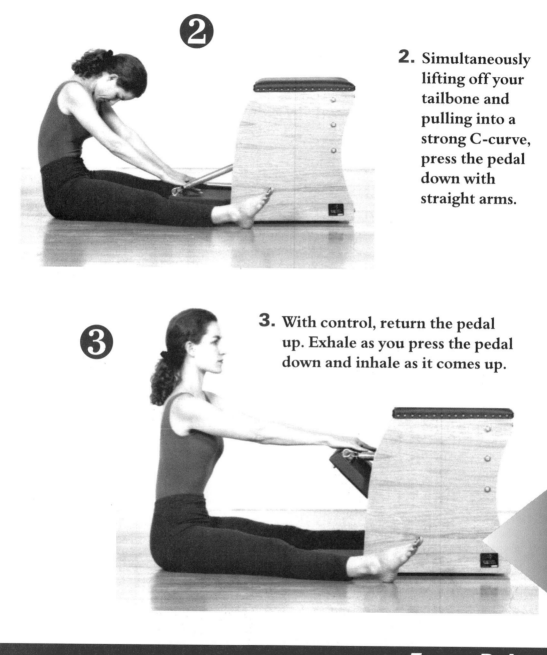

2. Simultaneously lifting off your tailbone and pulling into a strong C-curve, press the pedal down with straight arms.

3. With control, return the pedal up. Exhale as you press the pedal down and inhale as it comes up.

THE CHAIR

Focus Points

NOTE: This exercise is a great introduction to more advanced stretch and press exercises on the Chair.

Don't just sit down when pressing the pedal. Reach out of the pelvis and pull up, working into the C-curve.

Keep your arms as straight as possible and your shoulders down at all times.

Part 8

Special Exercise Routines

Pregnancy
Pre- and post-natal

Senior Citizens

Corrective Measures

Suggested Exercise Routines for Beginners

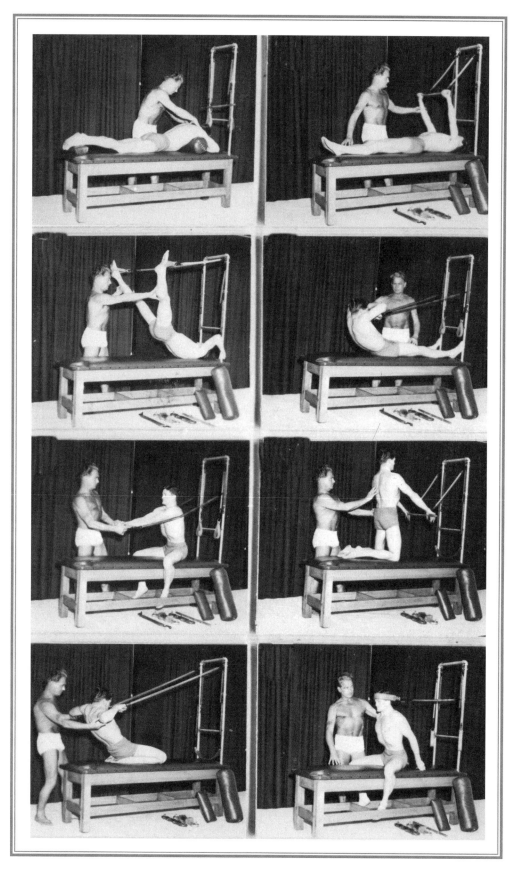

From the Pilates Archives

Pregnancy and Pilates Exercise

WARNING: Pilates is the perfect regimen to prepare your body for pregnancy and to remain flexible and strong while you are carrying. If you are not already training in the Pilates® Method prior to conception, it is not recommended that you begin after you become pregnant. However, the Method is ideally suited for postnatal recovery regardless of prior experience.

A pregnant woman undergoes an array of physiological changes during pregnancy which must be taken into consideration when formulating an exercise program. Pilates exercise helps to counter common pregnancy-related discomforts like backache, constipation, fatigue, bloating and swelling of the extremities. By increasing muscle tone, strength and endurance, it can also help with the physical stresses of pregnancy, especially carrying extra weight.

Women who were sedentary before becoming pregnant should start out with activities of a very low intensity and build up gradually. If a woman is not already exercising, she should build up to approximately three 30-minute sessions per week. Those who were exercising before pregnancy should be able to continue at the same level of intensity. The benefits of exercise during pregnancy require more study involving larger trials, but some of currently accepted advantages include:

- Maintains physical health and self-esteem.
- Fewer incidents of discomfort associated with pregnancy such as backache, constipation, shortness of breath, varicose veins, morning sickness and fatigue.
- Limited weight gain.
- Reductions in time in labor, the need for intervention and analgesia, and Cesarean section rates.

However, exercise isn't for every expectant mother. Women are advised to discuss participating in exercise during pregnancy with their primary caregiver. Any women with a history of miscarriages, placenta praevia, heart disease, severe toxemia, obesity, anemia, diabetes or thyroid disease are advised not to exercise during pregnancy.

For those women who have not participated in regular exercise, activities commonly prescribed during pregnancy include aerobic exercises, such as aqua-jogging, swimming, cycling and exercise to music classes. One reason these exercises are safer is that the risk of elevated body temperature is lessened at low to moderate exercise levels. Also low-impact exercise (such as Pilates) prevents the fetus from being subjected to the acidic waste products associated with anaerobic exercise such as sprinting and squash.

There are some basic precautions that any woman who is pregnant and wishes to exercise should take. In the first trimester nausea, vomiting and increased tiredness become daily obstacles. This may decrease the motivation to exercise. Elevated body temperatures above 102° F can occur with intensive exercise and may result in birth defects. If you keep your workouts to a moderate pace, you will escape the danger of raising your body temperature too high. In addition, you will not be intimidated by its rigor.

During pregnancy the hormone relaxin is

released to loosen the pelvis and all other joints in the body in preparation for childbirth. However, this increased joint laxity increases the potential for joint injury and muscular damage. No exercises should be executed one foot at a time (e.g. a single leg press), for this could harm the pelvic structure.

Many doctors advise not to lie on your back for too long as it may inhibit the mother's ability to efficiently deliver blood to the fetus. This view continues to cause controversy with some professionals. Pat Kupla, an obstetrician, believes such problems are not as common as implied and also gives the example of many women laboring on their backs.

Hypoglycemia is also considered a maternal risk of exercise. D. Hillis, in a 1990 study, considers both mother and baby at risk of premature labor as a result of this condition.

Activities that involve changes in pressure or high altitudes such as scuba diving or mountain climbing may affect oxygen supply to the baby, and should be generally considered off limits. Water skiing, trampolining, gymnastics and contact sports should also be avoided later in pregnancy.

Women are encouraged to listen carefully to their bodies. If they experience discomfort during exercise, the nature, duration or intensity of the exercise may need to be changed. The "talk test" is an indication of whether a woman is exercising at a safe level. If she is unable to talk, the exercise level is too intense. A recommended pulse rate is 140 beats per minute, but this is dependent on a women's previous heart rate and fitness level.

Other danger signs during pregnancy include:

- Any sign of blood discharge from the vagina.
- Any gush of fluid from the vagina.
- Persistent contractions (6-8/hour).
- Unexplained abdominal pain.
- Absence of fetal movement.
- Sudden swelling of ankles, hands and face.

- Persistent, severe headaches and visual disturbances.
- Unexplained spells of fainting or dizziness.
- Elevated pulse or blood pressure after exercise.
- Excessive fatigue, palpitations, and chest pain.
- Low weight gain in the last 6 months (2 lbs./month).

Any program should be developed on an individual needs basis and only after consultation with primary caregiver. Factors that could preclude a women from exercise and also danger signs should be discussed at that time.

References

Anderson, T. E., (1986). "Exercise and sport in pregnancy." *Midwife Health Visitor and Community Nurse*, 22 (8), 275-278.

Brody, Jane, et al. *The New York Times Book of Health*. New York. Random House.1997.

Clapp, J. F., (1989). "The effects of maternal exercise on early pregnancy outcome." *American Journal of Obstetrics and Gynecology*, 161 (6), 1453-1457.

Diploma in Sports Studies (1993). Exercise Testing and Prescription Paper, University of Otago.

Gauthier, M., (1986). "Guidelines for exercise during pregnancy: Too little or too much." *The Physician and Sports Medicine*, 14 (4), 162-169.

Highet, R. and Robyns, S., (1995). "Pregnancy and Exercise - a guide to safe exercise in pregnancy." Hillary Commission for Recreation and Sport Pamphlet.

Hillis, D., (1990). "Exercise during pregnancy." *Patient Management*, 19(6), 69-83.

Mittlemark, P. A., Wisewell, R. A. and Drinkwater, B. L., (1991). *Exercise in Pregnancy*. Baltimore: Williams and Wilkins.

Zeanah, M. and Schlosser, S. P., (1993). "Adherence to ACOG guidelines on exercise during pregnancy: Effect on pregnancy outcome." Journal of Obstetrics, Gynecologic and Neonatal Nursing, 22 (4), 329-335.

Pregnancy 1
Modified Roll-Up

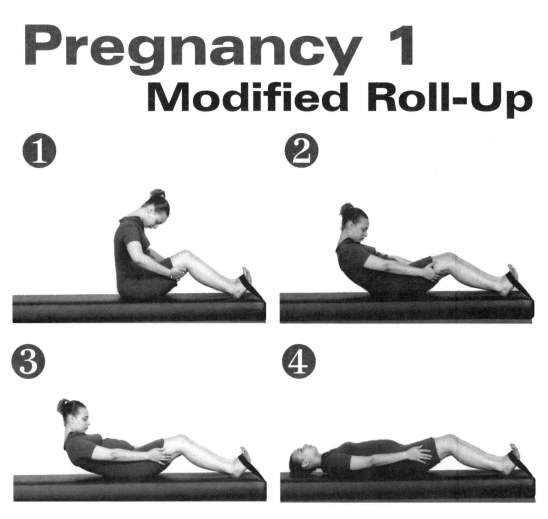

1. Start in the sitting position with your hands in the creases of the knees with the elbows bent. Your chin should be tucked down and pointed into the chest.

2. Roll back while holding onto your thighs as you straighten your elbows.

3. Continue rolling back while walking the hands up the thighs.

4. On the last repitition go all the way down to prepare for the Leg Circle. Do five repetitions.

Focus Points

In the last trimester most women will not be able to continue with this exercise.

Anchor your legs under a piece of furniture or have your partner hold your legs down.

The Pilates® Method

Pregnancy 2
Leg Circles

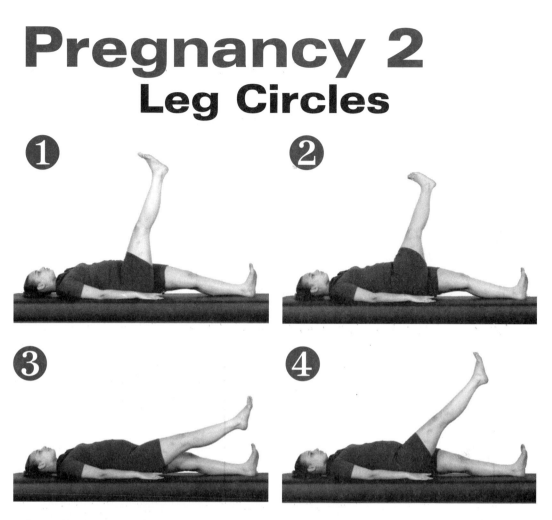

1. Lift the right leg up as high as possible while keeping the left flat and long against the mat.

2. Cross the right leg over the body.

3. Drop the right leg down until it is just above the left leg.

4. Bring the leg back to the right, in line with the torso, and then up and back to the starting position. Repeat 5 times, circle in the opposite direction 5 times and then do the exercise with the other leg.

Focus Points

Control must be maintained over the lifted leg and the pelvis at all times. Anchor one leg under a piece of furniture or have your partner hold one leg down.

Keep your hips steady. Make circle as large as you can control without wobbling.

Pregnancy 3
Single Leg Stretch

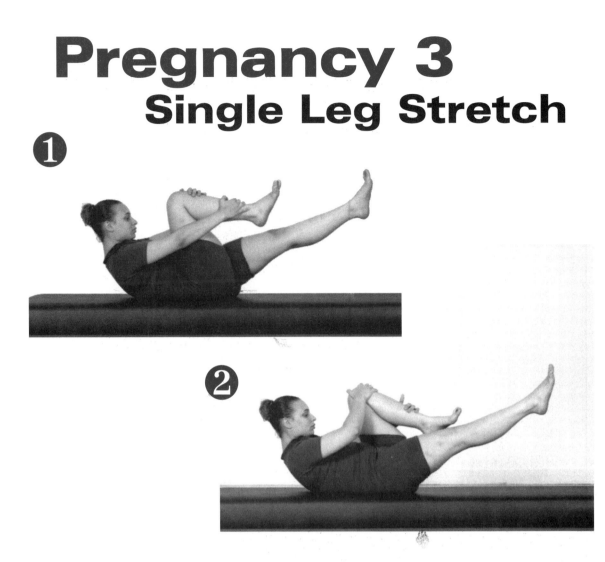

1. Pull your right leg towards you and bend it as far as possible towards your chest, inhaling slowly. Lift your chin to your chest. Place your left hand on your right knee and your right hand on your right ankle. This hand position is used to keep the ankle, knee and hip aligned.

2. Exhaling slowly, change legs and repeat with the left leg. Be sure to extend the right leg out. Repeat between 5 and 10 repetitions.

Focus Points

Women in the last trimester should avoid this exercise if they feel too much pressure in the stomach.

The Pilates® Method

Pregnancy 4
Double Leg Stretch

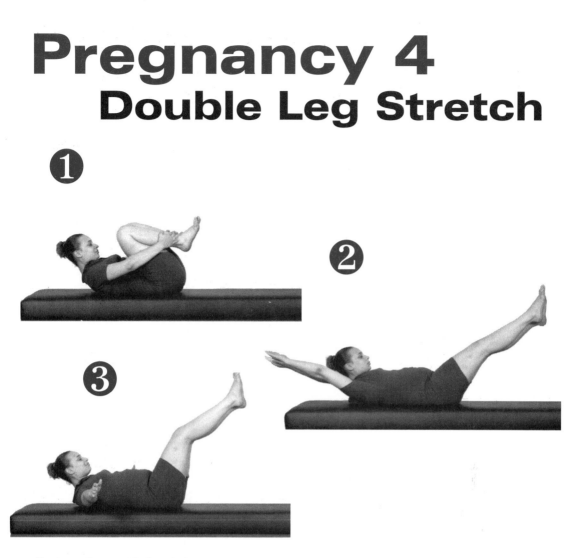

1. Lie flat with both legs bent into your chest. Pull your ankles in with your hands.

2. Inhaling slowly and keeping your chin in your chest, simultaneously reach overhead and point your legs out. Be sure to keep your stomach muscles in.

3. Exhaling slowly, circle your arms around and draw both legs upward into your chest again as shown in Step 1. Grab your ankles and hug your legs firmly to your chest while deepening the exhalation. Repeat 5 to 10 times.

Focus Points

Do not attempt to lower your legs any closer to the mat than you can maintain without strain. Women in the last trimester should avoid this exercise if they feel too much pressure in the stomach.

Do not use vigorous arm motions.

Pregnancy 5
Spine Stretch

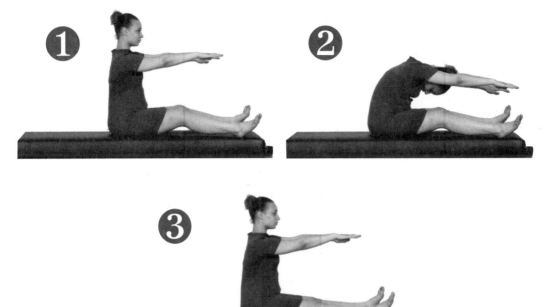

1. Sit with your legs straight and open slightly wider than shoulder width. Point your toes up. Extend your arms straight out at shoulder height.

2. Inhale and stretch your spine upwards moving from the head down. Chin pointing to your chest, roll down and forward. Keep your stomach muscles in and form a "C" with your lower back. Reach forward with a sliding motion. As the body stretches forward and down, keep the hip bones over the tailbone. Exhale.

3. On the inhalation, initiate from the navel and roll back up. Then sit up tall and exhale as seen in Step 1. Repeat 3 times and try to reach farther down and deeper into the spine with each repetition. Return to starting position.

Focus Points

In the last trimester most women will not be able to continue with this exercise

Bend forward and exhale gently.

The Pilates® Method

Pregnancy 6
Spine Twist

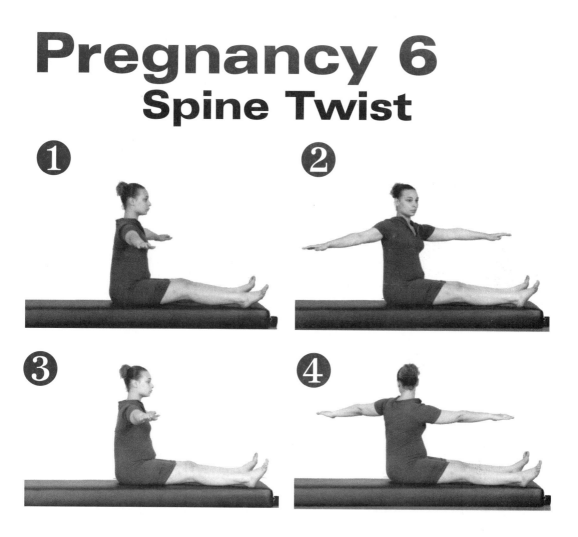

1. Sit up tall with your legs slightly wider than hip width apart. Extend the arms open to the sides. Draw the abdomen in.

2. Exhaling slowly, gently rotate your shoulders and twist your spine to the right at the waist (not the pelvis). Perform 3 "saw-like" pulses, stretching the waist. Complete the exhalation.

3. Initiating from the navel, return to the center.

4. Repeat three pulses to the left. Do 4 sets.

Focus Points

This exercise can be done standing up if sitting puts too much pressure on the stomach.

If you experience any pressure do not perform this exercise.

Pregnancy 7
Side Kick

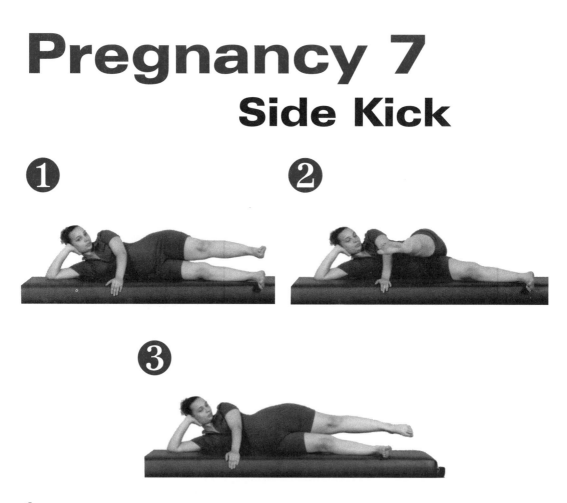

1. Lie on one side. Bend your bottom arm and support your head with your hand. Lie the full length, from hip to elbow, on the edge of the mat as shown. Place your opposite arm in front of your body to help support and keep your body in line. Lift the top leg to hip height. Keep the leg long and soft.

2. Inhaling slowly, swing the leg forward as far out as possible while maintaining the correct placement. Perform 2 pulses.

3. Exhaling slowly, swing the leg backward, reaching it as far behind the body as you can without shifting in the ribcage or in hip placement. Repeat a maximum of 10 times on each side.

Focus Points

Perform this exercise gently. Maintain navel to spine throughout.

Make sure that as you lift your leg up that you do not roll your hips forward or backward. A partner or trainer can stand behind you and gently press the hip in place.

The Pilates® Method

Pregnancy 8
Sitting and Squeezing

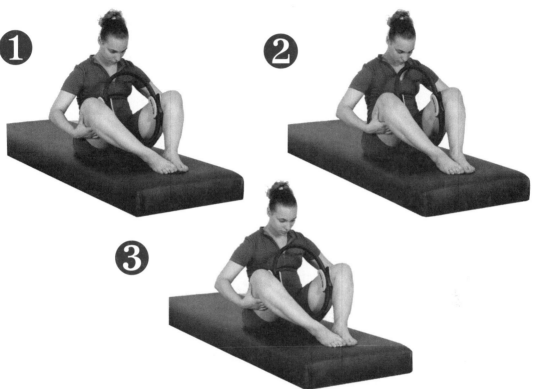

1. Start in the sitting position with your hands in the creases of the knees with the elbows bent and the Magic Circle or ball held between the lower thighs just above the knees. Your chin should be tucked down and into the chest.

2. Squeeze the Magic Circle or ball between the thighs for a count of three seconds.

3. Release and rest. Do 4 sets.

Focus Points

If you feel pressure anywhere do not perform this exercise.

Pregnancy 9
Rolling Down
with Squeezing

1. Start in the sitting position with your hands in the creases of the knees with the elbows bent and the Magic Circle or ball held between the lower thighs just above the knees. Your chin should be tucked down and into the chest.

2. Squeeze the the Magic Circle or ball between the thighs and roll back while holding onto your thighs as you straighten your elbows.

3. Continue rolling back while walking the hands up the thighs and maintaining the pressure on the Magic Circle or ball. Do 4 sets.

Focus Points

Have your partner hold your feet while performing this exercise.

The Pilates® Method

Suggested Exercises for Senior Citizens

There are senior citizens who are in excellent shape, some who suffer from a variety of nagging but non-threatening problems, and some who are in poor physical condition. Pilates can help many seniors regain muscle tone, improve posture, flatten the belly, alleviate some of the pain of arthritis and sciatica, improve breathing, and get the blood flowing to all parts of the body. Many seniors in their 60s, 70s, and 80s work out with the Pilates® Method.

Even if you are in excellent health and physical condition, we advise you to consult your physician before starting a new exercise program. You should also meet with a certified Pilates instructor to map out a targeted program for home use.

The following exercises in this book are suggested for senior citizens who have no serious health problems.

Single Leg Stretch, Exercise #4

This can be done on your bed or on a mat. Follow instructions on Page 38 except: Keep your leg up as high as possible. At the first sign of strain, lower the leg until you are comfortable.

Double Leg Stretch, Exercise #5.

This can be done on your bed or on a mat. Follow instructions on Page 40 except: Try to keep your head down without strain. Hold your hands on your legs instead of swinging them outward.

Spine Stretch Forward, Exercise #9.

This can be done on your bed or on a mat. Follow instructions on Page 48 except: Do not bend all the way forward and do not try to touch your feet. As you bend over, exhale.

The Wall: The Roll Down, Exercise #20.

Follow the instructions on Page 72 except: Bend over slowly and only until you feel the slightest strain. Stretch down toward your feet as much as possible.

Performer: Footwork 1-2: Exercises #44a and 44b.

Follow the instructions on Pages 128-131. Use heavy

socks or pads to protect your feet. Move gently. Place a pillow under your neck.

Performer: Stomach Massage & Round Exercise 51.

See Page 44. Perform Steps 1 and 2 only. Use a pad or heavy socks for your feet. Place a pillow under your neck.

The Chair: Arches: Exercise 63.

See Page 170. Place your toes on the bar. Do not use your arches. Place the chair against a wall so you can lean back against it for more comfort.   Use a pad or heavy socks to protect your feet.

Romana Kryzanowska's "TV Exercises" for Seniors

TV Shake: While watching television, during each commercial break, let your arms hang down and shake your hands and fingers for 20-60 seconds. Get the blood circulating. During the next break or commercial, raise your arms above your shoulders and shake your hands and fingers for 20-30 seconds.

Repeat as often as you can without strain. Rest for a while and repeat.

Leg Lift: Sit in your favorite chair as erect as possible. Pull your stomach in. Lift one leg straight up in the air as high as you can without strain. Hold it for three seconds. Lower your leg. Then lift the other leg and hold it straight up for three seconds. Stop when you feel any strain.

Squeeze the Ball: Here you perform an isometric exercise to tone your upper body. Imagine you are grabbing hold of a beach ball between your hands. Squeeze "the ball" and breathe deeply. Repeat as often as you are able.

Other Exercises in This Book

Once you feel comfortable with the exercises you have tried, you can move on to others in the book. A certified instructor can advise you which ones are appropriate. Mat exercises may require you to have a partner. Many Performer and Barrel exercises are good for seniors. Always read the Focus Points or warnings in each exercise. Avoid any exercise that can cause strain. Do not perform any Spring exercises without a certified Pilates instructor to assist.

All Pilates® Method exercises are corrective. The whole point of the Method is to stretch and strengthen the body while improving blood flow to all of its parts. Exercises massage and counter-massage the body parts, from the center to the extremities. If you have any major physical ailment, you must seek the advice of your doctor before beginning any regimen to improve or alleviate the symptoms. It is highly recommended to consult a certified Pilates instructor who can develop a program tailored to special physical problems.

BACK PAIN

Millions of people suffer from upper or lower back pain, mostly from poor body alignment and bad habits developed on the job. One of the hallmarks of the Pilates® Method is that back pain has been greatly alleviated. There are continuous testimonials from athletes, performers, business people, and others who have found relief, and many times, been cured from back pain. There is, of course, no guarantee that the Method can alleviate or cure all back pain. While virtually all Pilates exercises help the back, the following program is offered as a two-stage plan to bring relief.

STEP ONE

Perform the following exercises 2-3 times per week for a two-week period:
The Wall: Sitting on the Chair. Exercise #21 on Page 74. Do this exercise mildly at first with little strain.
The Wall Springs: Leg Circle. Exercise #23 on Page 80.
The Performer: Footwork 1-2. Exercises #44a & 44b on Pages 128-131.
The Performer: The Hundred. Exercise #45 on Page 132. Bend knees into chest and keep head on a pillow.
The Performer: Elephant. Exercise #50 on Page 142 .
The Performer: Stomach Massage: Round. Exercise #51 on Page 144.
The Performer: Running. Exercise #58 on Page 158.

STEP TWO:

In your third and fourth week, if your back has improved, repeat the first seven exercises in Step One and begin the following additional exercises:
The Wall: The Roll Down, Exercise #20 on Page 72.
Small Barrel or Small Pillow: Spine Corrector: Arm Circles, Exercise #37 on Page 112. Do not use the large barrel as shown in photographs. When using small barrel, place a pillow under your neck. Do not strain the neck backward.
The Performer: Stomach Massage: Hands Back, Exercise #52 on Page 146.
The Performer: Stomach Massage: Reach-Up, Exercise #53 on Page 148.
The Performer: Stomach Massage: Twist, Exercise #54 on Page 150.
Do steps one and two for a total of four weeks unless your back continues to cause pain. If improvement continues, you may move on with all the other Performer exercises.

OTHER PROBLEMS

Poor Posture: Follow the routines for the back exercises as they all align and strengthen the Powerhouse, which leads to correct and balanced posture. All exercises in this book will improve your posture and appearance, making you look lean and straight.
Love Handles and Flabby Buttocks: Every Mat exercise will help you firm your stomach and buttocks. See note on Page 14 about squeezing the buttocks. In addition to all the Mat exercises, the following Performer exercises will also help keep your body lean: #46, 47, 48, 49, 51, 52, 53, and 54.
Muscle & Joint Stiffness and Inflexibility: Every single Pilates exercise can relax stiff muscles and joints. If you are stiff, work the exercises cautiously, only doing as much as you can until you feel strain. As you become more flexible, pursue the exercises at will.
Tissue Damage: Consult a certified Pilates instructor who will devise a workable program for repair of soft tissue damage.

Exercise Routines for Beginners

If you do not wish to purchase the Performer apparatus, you can begin with the Mat exercises. Joseph H. Pilates started all of his clients on his Universal Reformer (found in Pilates Studios®). The Performer has been designed for inexpensive home use.

The Mat exercises are actually more difficult than the Performer, as the Mat requires you to fight against gravity and do all the work yourself. The Performer, using springs and straps, helps you do exercises more easily. Today's instructors believe that beginning with either the Mat or the Performer is challenging. If you begin with the Mat and want to complete the entire program, you will eventually need to purchase the Performer and other apparatus for home use.

The following routines are suggestions only, as very physically fit people may wish to perform more exercises in the beginning than those recommended; while people not in great physical shape may wish to lessen the number of exercises until they become adjusted to them.

OPTION ONE:

Beginning with the Mat and Working Toward all the Apparatus

Week One: The Mat

Work out three days, resting one day after each session.

> Day One: Perform the first 10 Mat exercises
>
> Day Two: Perform Mat exercises #11-19.
>
> Day Three: Perform all 19 Mat exercises.

Week Two: Mat, Magic Circle, Barrels

> Day One: Perform Mat exercises #1-19.
>
> Day Two: Perform Mat exercises #1-19, Wall Exercises #20-21; and Magic Circle exercises #33-34.
>
> Day Three: Perform all exercises and begin Barrel (Pillows) exercises #35,36, and 37.

Week Three: Review

> Days One, Two & Three: Perform all exercises learned so far.

Do not add any new exercise routines. Your goal this week is to gain skill on what you have learned and be able to move through the exercises gracefully without any jerkiness.

Week Four: Review & More Barrels

> Day One: Repeat all learned exercises.
>
> Day Two: Repeat all previous exercises and begin Barrel exercises #38, 39. and 40.
>
> Day Three: Repeat all previous exercises.

Week Five: Review & More Barrels

> Day One: Repeat all previous exercises.
>
> Day Two: Repeat all previous exercises and begin Barrel (Pillows) exercises #41, 42, and 43.
>
> Day Three: Repeat all exercises learned.

The Pilates® Method

NOTE: For the following weeks, you will need to purchase the Performer.

Week Six: Review & The Performer

Day One: Repeat all exercises and begin Performer exercises #44, 45, 46, 47, 49, and 49.

Day Two: Repeat all exercises learned.

Day Three: Repeat all exercises learned.

Week Seven: Review & More Performer

Day One: Repeat all exercises and begin Performer exercises #50, 51, 52, 53, and 54.

Day Two: Repeat all exercises.

Day Three: Repeat all exercises.

Week Eight: Review & More Performer

Day One: Repeat all exercises.

Day Two: Repeat all exercises and begin Performer exercises #55, 56, 57, 58, 59, and 60.

Day Three: Repeat all exercises.

Week Nine: Review

Day One: Repeat all exercises learned.

Day Two: Repeat all exercises.

Day Three: Repeat all exercises.

NOTE: By the end of Week Nine (or sooner if you are fitter) you will have learned all the core exercises on the Mat, Wall, Magic Circle, Barrels (Pillows), and Performer. The next routines require the use of the Wall Springs and the Chair. If you do not wish to purchase these apparatus, then merely repeat the exercises you have already learned 2-3 times per week. You can do some in the morning, some in the evenings, and some on weekends. The more you keep up with them, the better you will feel.

Week Ten: Review & Wall Springs

Day One: Repeat all exercises and begin Wall Springs exercises # 22, 23, 24, and 25. Remember, do not use Springs if you have bad knees. In the beginning, try to have a partner or certified instructor work with you.

Day Two: Repeat all exercises learned.

Day Three: Repeat all exercises.

Week Eleven: Review & More Springs

Day One: Repeat all exercises and begin Wall Springs #26, 27, 28. and 29.

Day Two: Repeat all exercises.

Day Three: Repeat all exercises.

Week Twelve: Review & More Springs

Day One: Repeat all exercises.

Day Two: Repeat all exercises and begin Wall Springs exercises #30, 31, and 32.

Day Three: Repeat all exercises

Week Thirteen: Review

Days One, Two and Three: Repeat all exercises.

Week Fourteen: Review & The Chair

Day One: Repeat all exercises and begin Chair exercises #61, 62, and 63.

Day Two: Repeat all and begin Chair exercises #64, 65 and 66.

Day Three: Repeat all exercises.

Week Fifteen and Onward:

You have now successfully completed the core exercises developed by Joseph H. Pilates. Congratulations! You now may simply continue with this program and gain skill and confidence with all the regimens. You may also contact your nearest Pilates instructor and work on additional exercises.

OPTION TWO:

Beginning with the Performer and Working Toward all other Apparatus.

Week One: The Performer

Work out three days, resting one day after each session.

Day One: Do Performer exercises #45 (Warm Up), 44a and 44b, 46, 47, and 48.

Day Two: Repeat exercises.

Day Three: Repeat exercises and begin Performer exercises #49, 50, 51, 52, 53, and 54.

Week Two: Performer

Day One: Repeat exercises learned.

Day Two: Repeat exercises and do Performer exercises #55, 56, 57, 58, 59, and 60.

Day Three: Repeat all exercises.

Week Three: Review

Days One, Two & Three: Execute all Performer exercises. Do not add any new exercise routines. Your goal this week is to gain skill on what you have learned and be able to move through the exercises gracefully without any jerkiness.

Week Four: Review, Wall & Magic Circle

Day One: Repeat all learned exercises.

Day Two: Repeat all previous exercises and begin Wall exercises #20 and 21.

Day Three: Repeat all previous exercises. Perform The Magic Circle exercises #33 and 34.

Week Five: Review

Day One: Repeat all previous exercises.

Day Two: Repeat all previous exercises and begin Barrels (Pillows) exercises #35, 36, and 37.

Day Three: Repeat all exercises learned.

Week Six: Review & More Barrels

Day One: Repeat all exercises and begin Barrel exercises #38, 39, and 40.

Day Two: Repeat all exercises learned.

Day Three: Repeat all exercises learned and begin Barrel exercises #41, 42 and 43.

Week Seven: Review & Mat

Day One: Repeat all exercises.

Day Two: Repeat all exercises and begin the first Mat exercises, #1 through 7.

Day Three: Repeat all exercises.

Week Eight: Review & More Mat

Day One: Repeat all exercises and begin Mat exercises #8 through 13.

Days Two and Three: Repeat all exercises.

Week Nine: Review & More Mat

Day One: Repeat all exercises learned.

Day Two: Repeat all exercises and begin Mat exercises #14 through 19.

Day Three: Repeat all exercises.

Week Ten: Review

Days One, Two and Three: Perform all exercises and gain confidence and skill.

NOTE: By the end of Week Ten (or sooner if you are fitter) you will have learned all the core exercises on the Performer, Wall, Magic Circle, Barrels (Pillows), and Mat. The next routines require the use of the Wall Springs and the Chair. If you do not wish to purchase these apparatus, then merely repeat the exercises you have already learned 2-3 times per week. You can do some in the morning, some in the evenings, and some on weekends. The more you keep up with them, the better you will feel.

Week Eleven: Review & Wall Springs

Day One: Repeat all exercises and begin Wall Springs exercises # 22, 23, 24, and 25. Remember, do not use Springs if you have bad knees. In the beginning, try to have a partner or certified instructor work with you.

Day Two: Repeat all exercises.

Day Three: Repeat all exercises.

Week Twelve: Review & More Springs

Day One: Repeat all exercises and begin Wall Springs #26, 27, 28. and 29.

Day Two: Repeat all exercises.

Day Three: Repeat all exercises.

Week Thirteen: Review & More Springs

Day One: Repeat all exercises.

Day Two: Repeat all exercises and begin Wall Springs exercises #30, 31, and 32.

Day Three: Repeat all exercises.

Week Fourteen: Review

Days One, Two and Three: Repeat all exercises.

Week Fifteen: Review & The Chair

Day One: Repeat all exercises and begin Chair exercises #61, 62, and 63.

Day Two: Repeat all and begin Chair exercises #64, 65 and 66.

Day Three: Repeat all exercises.

Week Sixteen and Onward:

You have now successfully completed the core exercises developed by Joseph H. Pilates. Congratulations! You now may simply continue with this program and gain skill and confidence with all the regimens. You may also contact your nearest certified Pilates instructor and work on advancing yourself further.

The website address: www.pilates-studio.com

This is a partial listing only. For up to date information contact The Pilates Studio

NEW YORK CITY
West Side
The Pilates Studio
2121 Broadway, Suite 201
New York, NY 10023
Sean P. Gallagher PT,
Director
(212) 875-0189
Fax: (212) 769-2368
Purchase Products
(888) 278-7227

East Side
Drago's Gym
50 West 57th Street 6th Fl.
New York, NY 10019
Romana Kryzanowska,
Master Teacher
(212) 757-0724
Sari Pace, Master Teacher

FLORIDA
Fort Myers
**The Pilates Studio
of Fort Myers**
11751 Cleveland Avenue
Ft. Myers, FL 33907
Hope Petrine, Director,
Certified Instructor
Suites 21 & 22
(941) 274-5711
Fax: 941-274-6622

ILLINOIS
Evanston
**The Pilates Studio of the
Midwest**
820 Davis Street, Suite 202
Evanston, IL 60201
Fatima Bruhns, Director,
Instructor
(847) 492-0464 Fax: 0210

WASHINGTON
Seattle
**The Pilates Studio of
Seattle & Capitol Hill
Physical Therapy**
413 Fairview Ave. North
Seattle, WA 98109
(206) 405-3560 Fax:3938
Lauren Stephen, Director,
Instructor
Lori Coleman Brown PT,
Director, Instructor

PENNSYLVANIA
Philadelphia
**The Pilates Studio @ the
P.A. Ballet**
1101 South Broad Street
Philadelphia, PA 19147
June Hines & Megan Egan
(215) 551-7000 x 1303
Fax: 7224

Bryn Mawr
**The Pilates Studio of Bryn
Mawr**
899 Penn Street
Bryn Mawr, PA 19010
Megan Egan, Director,
Instructor
(610) 581-0222 Fax: 610-
581-0223

GEORGIA
Atlanta
**The Pilates Studio @ the
Atlanta Ballet**
4279 Roswell Road, #703
Atlanta, GA 30342
Denise Reeves, Director
(404) 459-9555 Fax: (404)
459-9455

AUSTRALIA
Surry Hills
**The New York Pilates
Studio ® of Australia**
Director, Inst. Cynthia
Lochard.
Suite 12, Level 4/46-56
Tel / Fax: 011- 612- 9698-
4689
Instructors: Roula
Kantarzoglou,
Holt Street

Surry Hills, 2010 Australia
Edwina Ward
www.pilatesm.com

BRAZIL
The Pilates Studio
R. Cincinato Braga, 520
Tel/Fax: 011-551-1284-8905

Sao Paulo
Director/ Instructor, Inelia
Garcia
Bela Vista- Sao Paulo Brazil
Instructors: Robero Souza
Estevam,
ineliagarcia@hotmail.com
Cecilia Panelli Delgado

NETHERLANDS
**The New York Pilates
Studio of the Netherlands**

The Hague
Marjorie Oron, Instructor
Keizerstraat 32
Tel: 011 31 703 508 684

(BeNeLux)
Inst. Jane Poerwoatmodjo
2584 BJ The Hague,
Netherlands
Fax: 011 31 703 228285
e-mail: Marjorie@pilates.nl

ALABAMA
Gulf Shores
Misti McKee, Instructor
Tilawoop@zebra.net
Gulf Shores, AL 36542
(334) 955-6466

ALASKA
Fairbanks
Ann Turner, Instructor
621 Gingko Road
Fairbanks, AK 99709
aturner@mosquitonet.com
(907) 479-2360

ARIZONA
Phoenix
Fitness Solutions,
Inc.Lauren Tomasulo,
Owner, Instructor
4515 North 16th Street,
Suite 113
Phoenix, AZ 85016
Garry Rogers, Laura Talla
Instructors
(602) 631-9698

Phoenix
Pamela More, Instructor
Tel/Fax (602) 569-1612

Phoenix
Pamela LaPierre, Instructor
Phoenix, AZ 85008
(602) 817-4402

Phoenix
Tia Peterson, Instructor
t1window@earthlink.net
(602) 224-5220

Scottsdale
Studio Joe
Joey Greco, Instructor
7170 East McDonald , #5
Scottsdale, AZ 85253

Instructors: Sherry Brady
Greco,
(602) 367-8501
Janice Wessman, Pratibha
Noggle
(raventalks2@aol.com)

Scottsdale
Janice Wessman, Instructor
wessmanj@aol.com
Tel/Fax (602) 675-8501

Scottsdale
Harry Zabrocki, Instructor
Hzabro@aol.com
(602) 538-3046
Alicia Elliott, Instructor

Tuscon
John White, Instructor
2025 North Nancy Rose
Blvd
Tuscon, AZ 85712
(520) 319-8242

Tuscon
Suzanne Rosin, Instructor
7001 E. Eagle Point Place
Tuscon, AZ 85750
(520) 299-0544

Tuscon
Debi Crawford, Instructor
5451 N. Via Del Arbolito
Tuscon, AZ 85750
(520) 577-1597

CALIFORNIA
Alhambra
(South Pasadena)
Powerhouse
Sasha Koziak, Instructor
1003 Bushnell Street
Alhambra, CA 91801
Koziaks@pacbell.net
(626) 458-5600

Berkeley
Minoo Hamzavi , Instructor
1525 Spruce St. #36
Berkeley, CA 94709-1561
(510) 848-4133

Brea
Debra Noble, Instructor
dnoble@fullerton.edu.
Brea, CA 92821
(714) 671-4143

Above and Beyond Fitness
11601 Wilshire Blvd.
Brentwood, CA 90049

Brentwood
Sara Lovatt Carone,
Instructor
(310) 966-1999

Burbank
Merilee Blaisdell, Instructor
MerileeMB@aol.com
(818) 504-9630

Calabasas Hills
Jacqueline Berns,
Instructor,
(310) 317-0990

Carlsbad
Julia Hilleary, Instructor
(760) 431-7988
Carlsbad, CA 92009

Encino
Michael Levy Workout
Michael Levy, Instructor
17200 Ventura Boulevard,
#310
Encino, CA 91316
Instructors: Sara Lovatt
Carone
www.venturablvd.com/mich
ael-levy
(818) 783-0097

Hollywood
Bill & Jacqui Landrum
6315 Ivarene Avenue
Hollywood, CA 90068
jacquilandrum@earthlink.net
(323) 469-2012

West Hollywood
Valerie Von, Instructor
Vvon@msn.com
West Hollywood, CA 90046
(323) 850-6080

Irvine
(Orange County)
Audrey Wilson, Instructor
5 Bayberry Way
Irvine, CA 92612
(949) 551-3443
Audreydancing.com

West Los Angeles
It's A Stretch!
Linda Joy Luber, Instructor
jvert80774@aol.com
(310) 588-7376
Regina Fox Dawson,
Instructor

Los Angeles
Regina Fox Dawson,
Instructor
regdawson@yahoo.com
(310) 804-5663

Los Angeles
Licia Perea, Instructor
2159 Lyric Avenue
Los Angeles, CA 90027
(323) 669-3303
llperea@flash.net

Los Angeles
Jennifer Palmer, Instructor
(323) 394-5469

The Pilates® Method

Los Angeles
Susannah Todd, Instructor
Susannah13@aol.com
(818) 625-5488

Los Angeles
Niedra Gabriel, Instructor
616 N. Spaulding Ave.
Los Angeles, CA 90036
Karen Biancardi, Instructor
(323) 651-1796

Los Angeles
Charlene Hanson, Instructor
1745 Beloit Avenue #117
Los Angeles, CA 90025
(310) 312-8942

Los Angeles
Renda Mishalany
332 1/2 N. Orange Grove
Los Angeles, CA 90036
(213) 525-0293

Los Angeles
Miriam Kramer, Instructor
608 S. Dunsmuir Avenue
Los Angeles, CA 90036
Miriamkramer@yahoo.com
(323) 936-1369

Los Angeles
Laurel Canyon Studio
Heidi Kling, Instructor
8549 Walnut Drive
Los Angeles, CA 90046
(323) 654-4347 Fax: 2396

Los Angeles
Kara Springer, Instructor
kstw2000@gateway.net
Los Angeles, CA 90046
(323) 969-0475

Los Angeles
Nonna Gleyzer, Instructor
310 S. Hamel #103
Los Angeles, CA 90048
(310) 385-9485

Los Angeles
Karen Biancardi, Instructor
571 N. Gower
Los Angeles, CA 90004
(213) 957-2035

Los Angeles
Geoffrey Rhue, Instructor
1435 Bellevue Ave
Los Angeles, CA 90026
(213) 926-3588

Lomita/Torrance
Joellyn Musser, Instructor
24725 Pennsylvania Ave. C-19
Lomita, CA 90717
(310) 530-7881
clbr8lif@earthlink.net

Malibu
Survival of the Fittest
Jacqueline Berns,
Instructor, Owner
3806-J Cross Creek Rd
Malibu,CA 90265
(310) 317-0990

Malibu
Phyllis Reffo, Instructor
30125 Harvester Road
Malibu, CA 90265
(310) 457-8751

Newport Beach
BodyFit
Sheena Jongeneel, Owner,
Instructor
3422 Via Lido
Newport Beach, CA 92663
Anna Caban, Instructor
(949) 675-2639

Newport Beach
Anna Caban, Instructor
newbody246@yahoo.com
Newport Beach, CA 92663
(949) 246-BODY

North Hills
Sarah Lovatt-Carone,
Instructor
9219 Hagvenhurst Ave
North Hills, CA 91344
(818) 893-5387

Oakland
Katherine Davis, Instructor
KDavis5267@aol.com
Oakland, CA 94610
(510) 832-0653

Ojai
Mary Jo Healy, Instructor
218 North Padre Juan Ave
Ojai, CA 93023
Jinny Feiss, Instructor
(805) 646-3797
healy@ojai.net
Fax: (805) 640-8930

Orange County
Lisa May Costich, Instructor
Lisamay98@hotmail.com

Pasadena
ZOE
Zoe Hagler, Owner /
Instructor/ Teacher Trainer
21 South El Molino
Pasadena, CA 91101
Instructors: Geoffrey Rhue,
Merilee Blaisdell
(626) 585-8853
Susannah Todd, Danielle
Marcus Janssen, Lara
Serventi

Pasadena
Rachel Bhagat, Instructor
rbhagat1@hotmail.com

Redondo Beach
Arlene Renay Reese,
Instructor
313 Avenue G
Redondo Beach, CA 90277
(310) 540- 5539

San Diego
Studio Mo
Moses Urbano, Instructor
studiomo@home.com
San Diego, CA 92103
(619) 295-1850
Fax: (619) 295-1023

San Francisco
Golden Gate Studio
3209 Pierce Street
San Francisco CA
Lucero Barry, Instructor
(415) 637-7919

San Francisco
Catherine Kirsch, Instructor
(415) 288-1001 X 7064
Cherrie_34@hotmail.com

San Francisco
Kerri Palmer Gonen,
Instructor
kp_trainer@yahoo.com
San Francisco, CA 94131
Fax: (415) 441-6985

San Francisco
Nancy Rosellini, Instructor
387 Staples Ave
San Francisco, CA 94112
(415) 441-6985

San Francisco
Jennifer Palmer, Instructor
4135 Cesar Chavez, #14
San Francisco, CA 94131

Santa Monica
Nela Fry, Instructor
1008 Euclid Street
Santa Monica, CA 90403
Tel / Fax (310) 394-2805
nela@csi.com

Santa Monica
Heather Leon, Instructor
508A Santa Monica Blvd
Santa Monica, CA 90401
(310) 394-9780

Santa Monica
April Howser, Instructor
Aprilhowser@hotmail.com
Santa Monica, CA 90401
(310) 434-9130

Santa Monica
Jennifer Bocian, Instructor
(310) 260-9736

Sebastopol
Watta Lee-Ribas, Instructor
613 Sparkes Rd.
Sebastopol , CA 95472
birthrites@igc.org
(707) 823-2879

Sherman Oaks
The Body Coach
Susan Lonergan, Instructor
(818) 905-6856

Sherman Oaks
Courtney, Ca Instructor
coure@att.net
(818) 986-8361

Sherman Oaks
Trish Garland Studio
13803 Ventura Blvd.
Sherman Oaks, CA 91423
Trish Garland, Instructor
(818) 385-0012
trish_garland@hotmail.com

Studio City
The Gold Touch
11333 Moorpark Street,
#402
Studio City, CA 91602
Darien Gold, Instructor
(888) 908-4778

West Hollywood
Winsor Fitness
Mari Winsor, Instructor
945 North LaCienega
West Hollywood, CA 90069
(310) 289-8766 Fax: 0812

Westlake Village
Deborah Mandis Cozen,
RPT, Instructor
3034 Winding Lane
Westlake Village, CA 91361
(805) 373-1030

Westwood
Adylia Roman, Instructor
Westwood, CA 90024
(310) 446-6100 fax: 1128

COLORADO
Boulder
Flatiron Athletic Club
Deidre Szarabajka,
Instructor
505 Thunderbird Drive
Boulder, CO 80301
Michelle Perkins, Instructor
(303) 499-6590
emmaandmichelle@yahoo.com

Breckenridge
Jessica Paffrath, Instructor
Breckenridge, CO 80424
(970) 453-2139

Denver
Amy Halaby, Instructor
(Denver Athletic Club)
Denver, CO 80204
1325 Glenarm Place
(720) 931-6743
Body & Mind Awareness

Engelwood
Carlye Flom, Instructor
Engelwood, CO 80111
(303) 221-5012

CONNECTICUT
Bridgeport
Monica Mauri, Instructor
Bridgeport, CT 06605
(203) 333-8926

Cos Cob
Terese Garsson, Instructor
14 Pond Place
Cos Cob, CT 06807
(Near Greenwich &
Stamford)
Tgarsson@aol.com
(203) 629-5543

Colebrook
Eliot Foote, Instructor
Colebrook, CT 06021
(860) 379-9982

Greenwich
Pure Pilates
Mejo Wiggin,
Owner/Instructor
(203) 629-3743
Instructors: Wendy Oliver,
Molly Niles, Junghee
Kallander

Greenwich
Patricia Erickson, Instructor
P.O Box 7737
Greenwich, CT 06836
Tel / Fax (203) 661-1848
pattyerick@aol.com

CONNECTICUT
Greenwich
Glynis Bylciw, Instructor
(203) 622-1793

New Cannan
The Movement Place
Holly Mensching, Instructor
11 Burtis Avenue
New Cannan, CT 06840
Cameron Buday, Instructor
(203) 972- 3438

New Haven
Lenore Frost,CHT, OTR/L ,
Instructor
61 Amity Road, Suite B
New Haven, CT 06515
(203) 389-8177

Norfolk
Sarah Smolen, Instructor
(860) 542-0081

Norwalk
Oleg Belousou, Instructor
(203) 847-0591

Ridgefield
Simone Wunderli-Rucolas,
Instructor
124 Tanton Hill Rd
Ridgefield, CT 06877
(203) 438-7984
Swisssimi@aol.com

South Norwalk
Amy Matton, Instructor
South Norwalk, CT 06854
(203) 831-8701

Thomaston
Jeffrey Smolen, Instructor
(860) 283-6428

Westport
Bodywork Studio
Instructors: Cristina Bruno
645 Post Road East
Westport, CT 06880
Lynn Bartner, Ossi Raveh,
Jeanne Turkel
(203) 226-8550 Fax: 222-
0731

Westport
Womens Fitness Edge
Caroline Benton, Instructor
(203) 454-3343
Fax: (203) 454-3342

Westport
Lynn Bartner , Instructor
LMB21665@AOL.COM

West Hartford
Elizabeth Flores, Instructor
41 South Main Street
West Hartford, CT 06107
(860) 233-5232

FLORIDA
Boca Raton
The Balanced Body Inc.
Cecil SY Ybanez, PT,
Instructor
5580 N. Federal Highway
Boca Raton, FL 33487
(561) 994-8848

Boca Raton
Boca Body Works
7088 Beracasa Way
Boca Raton, FL 33433
Cindy Maybruck, Instructor
cmaybruck@aol.com
(561) 347-1110
Fax: 561-395-7544

Burnell
Robin Campbell, Instructor
(904) 437-6022

Delray Beach
John Mahoney, Instructor
39 Gleason Street
Delray Beach, FL 33483
(561) 703-5646

Deerfield Beach
Linda Collier, Instructor
820 SE 14th Street
Deerfield Beach, FL 33441

Fort Lauderdale
Alternative Training Studio
David Freeman, Instructor
1517 S.E. Second Street
Fort Lauderdale, FL 33301
AlternativeTS@aol.com
(954) 764-2248

Fort Lauderdale
Martha (Marty)
Hammerstein
516 SW 12th Court
Fort Lauderdale, FL 33315
(954) 525-8565

Fort Myers
**The Pilates Studio
of Fort Myers**
11751 Cleveland Avenue
Ft. Myers, FL 33907
Hope Petrine, Director,
Certified Instructor
Suites 21 & 22
(941) 274-5711
Fax: 941-274-6622
Melissa Derstine, Instructor

Miami
Alba Calzada Carter,
Instructor
175 NE 96th Street
Miami, FL 33138
(305) 757-0440

Orlando
**Jacki Garland Studio Mod
Bod 2000**
5891 Tradewinds Lane
Orlando, FL 32819
Instructors: Jacki Garland,
Jessica Gazzola,
Samantha Gazzola
(407) 903-0641

Palm Beach County
Catherine Cuzzone,
Instructor
cmcinri@aol.com

St. Petersburg
Movement In Motion
Linda McNamar, Instructor
1833-9th Street North
St. Petersburg, FL 33704
(727) 822-4722

St. Petersburg
Angela Zaun, Instructor
5655 A Lynn Lakes Drive
South
St. Petersburg, Fl 33712

Sarasota
Dynamic Fitness Inc.
Sherry Resh, Instructor
4141 South Tamiami Trail
Sarasota, FL 34231
Instructors: Isa Lambert,
Suite 11
(941) 929-9885
S.Resh@aol.com
Christina Bladon

Winter Park
The Bougainvillea Clinique
Michelle Hartog, R.N.,
Instructor
4355 Bear Gully Rd
Winter Park, FL 32792
mglowhart@aol.com
(407) 678-3116

Winter Park
MatWorkz
Debra Watson, Instructor
558 W. New England Ave
Ste. 200
Winter Park, FL 32789
April Aubiel, Instructor
www.matworkz.com
(407) 628-4888

GEORGIA
Atlanta
**The Pilates Studio @ the
Atlanta Ballet**
4279 Roswell Road, #703
Atlanta, GA 30342
Denise Reeves, Instructor,
Director
(404) 459-9555
Instructors: Robin Warden,
Deidra Simon, Jamie Trout,
Emily Bradley, Edgar Tirado,
Lisa Browning
Doris Van Glahn

Atlanta
Body Central
3005 Peachtree Road
Atlanta, GA 30305
Penelope Wyer, Director,
Instructor
Suite 200
(404) 233-3656
Instructors: Leah
Rutkowski, Amy Kopala,
Fax: (404) 266-2103
Cristine Williams, Jamie
Trout, Kelly Beasley,
Christina Peene, Liz Elliot,
Robin Warden, Amanda
Lower

Atlanta
Studio Lotus
Flo Fitzgerald, Director,
Instructor
1145 Zonolite Road Suite 13
Atlanta, GA 30306
Nikki Regent, Alysha
Oclassen,
www.studiolotus.com
(404) 817-0900
Robin Warden, Emily
Bradley, Heather King
Elizabeth Purdy

Atlanta
Alysha Oclassen, Instructor
Alyho@aol.com
Atlanta, GA 30308
(678) 592-6601

Decatur
Regina Christler, Instructor
3828 Kensingwood Trace
Decatur, GA 30032
(404) 298-5844

Duluth
Elizabeth Elliott, Instructor
Lelliott2@aol.com
(678) 624-7552

Marietta
Core Bodyworks
1355 Church Street Ext.
Marietta, GA 30060

Marietta
Lisa Browning, Instructor
LBSMT@aol.com
(770) 231-7849

Norcross
The Work
5952 Peachtree Ind. Blvd.
Norcross, GA

Edgar Tirado, Instructor
Ste. #16
(770) 518-9610

HAWAII
Pukalani
Belkis Lozada, Instructor
Belkis@mauigateway@aol.c
om
Pukalani, HI 96788

IDAHO
Boise
Forte
Carrie Shanafelt, Instructor
222 North 10th
Boise, ID 83702
Forteboise@earthlink.net
(208) 342-4945

INDIANA
Muncie
Positive Movement
1411 West Red Maple Road
Muncie, IN 47303-9314
June Hutchinson, Instructor
juneh@hr.cami3.com
(765) 288-5116

ILLINOIS
Antioch
Patricia L. Kendziora
Antioch, IL
(847) 395-2686

Barrington
Welcome to Your Body, Inc.
Maryanne Radzis, Instructor
220 S. Cook Street
Barrington, IL 60010
(847) 304-4900

Barrington
Susan Hacker, Instructor
(773) 489-9844

Bloomingdale
Craig Franzen, Instructor
Bloomingdale, IL 60108
(630) 529-0120

Chicago
Stacy Weitzner, Instructor
(773) 529-7104

Chicago
Juanita Lopez, Instructor /
Teacher Trainer
(312) 878-3639

Chicago
Julie Schiller, Instructor
1016 N Dearborn
Chicago, IL 60610
(773) 871-2385

Chicago
Integrations, Inc.
Kevin Bradley, Instructor
1111 North Dearborn,
#1905
Chicago, IL 60610
(312) 280-7950 &8944

Chicago
David Englund, Instructor
1912 Lincoln Park West
Chicago, IL 60714
(312) 932-0991
Mrerolfu@aol.com

Chicago
**Chiropractic Health
Resources**
Instructors: Ceci Fano-
Bryan,
2105 N. Southport #208
Chicago, IL 60614
Jacqueline Brenner, Corrine
Stanislaw
(773) 472-0560
Linda Spriggs

Chicago
Therese Stark, Instructor
Chicago, IL 60614
(773) 327-4341

Chicago
**Body Endeavors-
Performance Gym**
1000 West North Ave. 3rd Fl.
Chicago, IL 60622Liv
Berger, Instructor
Lsbodydesign@1box.com
(312) 202-0028
Fax: (312) 751-8122

Chicago
Gail Tangeros, Instructor
1720 West Leland #2
Chicago, IL 60640
gtangeros@ameritech.net
(773) 561-2854

Chicago
Krista Merrill, Instructor
5030 N Parkside Ave
Chicago, IL 60630
(773) 545-6165

Chicago
Susan Hacker, Instructor
(773) 489-9844

Chicago
**Fitness Foundations
Chicago**
213 West Institute Place,
#303
Chicago, IL 60610
Instructors: Linda Tremain
(312) 642-5633 Fax: 5733
Krista Merrill, Juliet Cella
ltremain@sprynet.com

Chicago
Erin Harper, Instructor
5313 N. Ravenswood, #301
Chicago, IL 60640
(773) 989-9979

Chicago
**The Pilates Studio of the
Midwest at Hubbard Dance
Complex**
1151 West Jackson Ave.
Chicago, IL 60607
(312) 492-8835
Dana Santi -Manager, Instr.
Fax: (312) 492-8875
Instructors: Joe Palla,
Julie Dewerd, P.T.
Jill Domke

Chicago
**The Pilates Studio of the
Midwest**
185 N. Wabash
Chicago, IL 60601
at Ballet Chicago

Chicago
Joe Palla, Instructor
5828 N. Paulina
Chicago, IL 60660
(773) 334-6491

Dundee
Kimberly Jerrick, Instructor
Dundee, IL 60118
(847) 428-6143

Evanston
The Pilates Studio of the Midwest
820 Davis Street, Suite 202
Evanston, IL 60201
Fatima Bruhns, Director
(847) 492-0464 Fax: 0210

Evanston
Cheryl Ivey, Instructor
1723 Benson
Evanston, IL 60201

Evanston
Christine Pickering,
Instructor
Cepicke@attglobal.net

Evanston
Patricia Medros, Instructor
Hwg2948@aol.com
Evanston, IL 60201
(847) 491-6304

Evanston
Lady Holly Hathaway,
Instructor
2147 Sherman Avenue #3,
Evanston, IL 60201
(847) 864-4318

Glen Carbon
(St. Louis Area)
The Integrated Body
Pam Moody, Instructor
23-C Kettle River Drive
Glen Carbon, IL 62034
(618) 656-3890

Glenview
Loribeth Cohen, Instructor
3122 Crestwood Lane
Glenview, IL 60025
(847) 998-5859 or (847)
624-7455

Highland Park
In Synch Fitness Corp.
1898 First Street
Highland Park, IL 60035
Fatima Bruhns, Director,
Inst.
(847) 266-1512
Instructors: Debbie
LaMantia, Randi Neebe, Joe
Palla
Patty Kendziora, Allegra
Love

Lake Villa
Cathie Derer- McCue,
Instructor
38569 Route 59
Lake Villa, IL 60046
(near border of WI)
(847) 356-0180
CDM _HEALTHY_ BODY @
Juno.com

NorthShore
Cheryl Ivey, Instructor
NIY1BERGIE@aol.com
(847) 651-5413

Oakbrook
Fitness Foundations, Inc.
Instructors: Linda Tremain
1111 West 22nd Street, #610
Oakbrook, IL 60523
Jill Popovich, Amy
McDowell, Krista Merrill
(630) 573-5877 Fax: 5875
Erin Harper
ltremain@sprynet.com

Oak Park
Alternative Fitness Studio
126 N. Oak Park Ave
Oak Park, IL 60302
Andrea Andrade, Instructor
(708) 386-4930

Skokie
Barbara Wertico, Instructor
8728 N. Drake
Skokie, IL 60076
(847) 677-7573
BarbWertico@compuserve.com

Skokie
Barbara Stoltz, Instructor
(847) 677-3194

St. Charles
Total Body Dynamics, Inc.
Kim Jerrick, Instructor
2049 Lincoln Highway
St. Charles, IL 60174
630-584-2790

Willowbrook
Dana Santi, Instructor
6141 Knoll Wood Rd
Willowbrook, IL 60514
DanaST919@aol.com
(630) 654-9834

IOWA
Bettendorf
Gail Diehl, Instructor
4640 Crow Creek Court
Bettendorf, IA 52722-6925
(319) 332-8625

KANSAS
Overland Park
Modern Body Contrology
David Mooney, Instructor
9308 Dearborn
Overland Park, KS 66207
(913) 649-1479 Fax: same

Olathe
Leslie Johnson, Instructor
(716) 638-5157

LOUISIANA
New Orleans
Larry Gibas, Instructor
Whenandif@aol.com
New Orleans, LA 70115
(504) 862- 6210

New Orleans
Monica Noriega Wilson,
Instructor
Bwilson@mailhost.tcs.tulan
e.edu
(504) 894-1665

MAINE
Sustainable Fitness
96 Main Street
Belfast, ME 04915

Belfast
Beth Tracy, Instructor
(207) 338-2977

Camden
Maureen (Mo) Freeman,
Instructor
133 Washington Street
Camden, ME 04843
maureen@mint.net
(207) 230-0073

Portland
Body Balance
49 Portsmouth Street
Portland, ME 04107
Nancy Etnier, Instructor
(207) 772-8950

Rockland
Ily Shofestall, Instructor
The Thorndike
Rockland, ME 04841
385 Main Street
(207) 596-6177

MASSACHUSETTS
Boston
(Back Bay)
Progressive Bodyworks
Clare Dunphy-Foster,
Instructor
441 Stuart Street
Boston, MA 02116
(617) 247-8090
Vania Nabuco Sacramento,
Sarah Faller, Kyra Strasberg
strongbody@aol.com

Boston
Sarah Faller, Instructor
Boston, MA
(617) 269-4300 x187

Cambridge
Green Street Studio's
Martha Mason, Instructor
185 Green Street
Cambridge, MA 02139
Lisa Silveira, Instructor
(617) 491-2940

Gloucester
Joe Porcaro, Instructor
Gloucester, MA 01930
(978) 283-4531

Lenox
Uli Nagel, Instructor
(888) 969-6668
Fitness Finesse Inc.

North Weymouth
Cheryl Lathum, Instructor
North Weymouth, MA
(781) 736-0000

Salem
Jimmy Raye, Instructor
21 Salem Street
Salem, MA 01970
(978) 741-1540

Stockbridge
Mathilde M. Klein, P.T., Inst.
21 South Street, Box 1219
Stockbridge, MA 01262
(413) 298-3896

Wakefield
**Flexfit Mind &
Body Training Center**
Carla Dunlap-Kaan,
Instructor, Owner
607 N. Avenue, Door 14
Wakefield, MA 01880
(781) 245-9143
coccobuns@carladunlap.com

MARYLAND
Baltimore
Goucher College
Instructors: Elizabeth Lowe
Ahearn,
1021 Dulaney Valley Road
Baltimore, MD 21204-2794
Linda R. Moxley, Lynne
Balliette, Julie Clime,
Jennifer Ellsworth
(410) 337-6399 Fax: 6433
eahearn@goucher.edu

Hagerstown
Diane Popper, Instructor
Snowkysp@msn.com
(301) 745-4118 or (301)
991-8343

Frederick
Linda Rinier Moxley,
Instructor
(301) 694-3015

Mount Rainer
Michael Rooks, Instructor
Rookery@worldnet.att.net
(301) 927-5127

Mount Rainer
Andrea Chastant, Instructor
achastant@att.net
(301) 927-2134

Towson
Lynne Balliette, Instructor
269 Ridge Avenue
Towson, MD 21286
lballiet@goucher.edu
410-337-6531 x 1

MICHIGAN
Detroit
Wayne State University
Theatre Dept.
4841 Cass Ave, Suite 3225
Detroit, MI 48202
Nira Pullin, Instructor
(313) 577-3508
(612) 672-6697
**(For Univ. Theatre Students
Only)**

MISSOURI
Columbia
In Line Studio
Janice Dulak, Owner,
Instructor
Studio located on
Stephens College Campus
Columbia, MO
Amy Higgins-Stambaugh,
Instructor
(573) 442-2211 x4715 (Studio)
(573) 449-0583 (Business)
Ahstambaugh@hotmail.com

(St. Louis Area)
Pam Moody, Instructor
340 South Fillmore
Edwardsville, IL 62025
(618) 692-9763

Kirkwood
Susan Bronstein, Instructor
11830 Big Bend Road
Kirkwood, MO 63122
(314) 965-5672 Fax: 9317

NEW JERSEY
Absecon
Holly's Dance & Body Arts
Holly Bozzelli, Instructor
119 Marin Drive
Absecon, NJ 08201
(near Atlantic City)
(609) 383-8822

Clifton
Karen Schoenberger,
Instructor
Karsch@ix.netcom.com
(973) 779-7116

Englewood Cliffs
Hedy Weisbart, Instructor
HLW3@aol.com
(201) 567-8763

Englewood
Jeannie Lee, Instructor
Englewood, NJ 07670
(201) 568-0425

Haledon
Julie LoRusso, Instructor
gary-julie@worldnet.att.net
(973) 790-4243

Hohokus
Body Tech
Kathryn Ross-Nash,
Instructor
500 Barnett Place
HoHokus, NJ 07423
bodytech@pipeline.com
(201) 444-6200

Kingston
Integrated Fitness
Donna C. Longo, Instructor
4595 Route 27
Kingston, NJ 08528
POB 44
(609) 252-9229 &
(609)252-0997

Milltown
Tori Sikkema, Instructor
Tori@debiz.com
Milltown, PA 08850
(Counties: Monmouth,
Ocean & Mercer)
(609) 538-4420

Princeton
Anthony Rabara, Instructor
377 Wall Street
Princeton, NJ 08540
(609) 921-7990

Princeton Junction
Marie Snyder, Instructor
Marie-snyder@iname.com
(609) 918-9365

Red Bank
Reform Studio
30 W. Front Street
Red Bank, NJ 07701
Kim Lauda, Instructor
(732) 212-0700

Ridgewood
Arlene Dodd, Instructor
75 Wilson Street
Ridgewood, NJ 07450
(201) 445-3102

Teaneck
Lisa Gratale, Instructor
Energybodystudio@aol.com
Teaneck, NJ 07666

Titusville
Zane Rankin, Instructor
50A River Drive
Titusville, NJ 08560
(609) 730-9544

Upper Montclair
The Movement Place
Instructors: Holly
Mensching, Karen Cooper &
Karin Schoenberger,
Cameron Buday
48 Northview Avenue
Upper Montclair, NJ 07043
(973) 746-2577

Waldwick
Pamela DeJohn, Instructor
51 Waldwick Avenue
Waldwick, NJ 07463
pamdej@wordnet.att.net
(201) 652-5986

Westmont
Donna M. Tambussi,
Instructor
20 Haddon Avenue
Westmont, NJ 08108
(856) 869-3569

NEW MEXICO
Santa Fe
Kathleen Loeks, Instructor
615 Calle de Leon
Santa Fe, NM 87505
kloeks@cybermesa.com
(505) 984-2909
Fax:(505) 982-7411

Santa Fe
Stacy Weitzner, Instructor
Awgalt@worldnet.att.net
(505) 988-4489

NEW YORK STATE
Albany
Body Wisdom
Ellen A. Weinstein,
Owner/Instructor
344 Fuller Road
Albany, NY 12203
(518) 435-1064

Albany
Jeanette Sommer,
Instructor
Jette16@Juno.com
Albany, NY 12203
(518) 456-3884

Bayside
Firm "n" Flex
Theresa Familio, Instructor
(917) 919-2522 or (516)
524-0156

Bedford
Vandy Lipman, Instructor
66 Millbrook Road
Bedford, NY 10506
(914) 234-6079

Briarcliff Manor
(Westchester County)
Saro Vanasup,
Owner/Instructor
(914) 762-0040

Brooklyn
(Park Slope)
Jessica Fadem, Instructor
(718) 469-2265

Brooklyn
(Park Slope)
BodyTonic
Jennifer DeLuca, Instructor
150 5th Avenue
Brooklyn, NY 11215
(718) 622-2755

Brooklyn
Metta Coleman, PT,
Instructor
(Mount Sinai Hospital, NYC)
Metira@aol.com

Brooklyn
Brooklyn Body Control
Rosanna Barberio,
Instructor
177 Smith St. Grnd Floor
Brooklyn, NY 11201
(718) 246-2447

Brooklyn
Tiziana Trovati, Instructor
(718) 722-7886

Brooklyn
Elizabeth Stile, Instructor
(718) 636-5113

Brooklyn
(Prospect Heights)
Ali Daniels, Instructor
(718) 638-8334

Centerport
Terri Safaii, Instructor
(631) 757-5441

Cold Spring Harbor Amy
Wilson, Instructor
(516) 815-5505

Fishers Island
Susan Connelly, Instructor
PO Box 648
Fishers Island, NY 06390
(516) 788-7750

Flushing
Sonia D. Orevillo, Instructor
Soniadomor@aol.com
Flushing, NY 11354
(718) 321-9069

Great Neck
(Long Island)
Fitness Studio at Marathon
Doug Pollack, PT,
Instructor / Owner
330 Great Neck Road
Great Neck, NY 11021
Instructors: Theresa
Familio, Linda Figlia
(516) 829-2938

Great Neck
Total Body Dynamics
(516) 944-0670
Patricia O'Donnell,
Instructor

Greenlawn
Mary Lundy Studio
Mary Lundy, Instructor
46 Fenwick Street
Greenlawn, NY 11740
(516) 757-9050

Glen Cove
Charmian Surface,
Instructor
Glen Cove, NY 11542
(516) 671-3912

Hastings On Hudson
Bodyscape
Kerry Donegan, Instructor
5 Boulanger Plaza
(914) 478-2639

Huntington
(Long Island)
**Maggie Amrhein's Exercise
Studio**
Maggie Amrhein, Owner
15 Green St
Huntington, NY 11743
Instructors: Teri Safaii,
Amy Wilson
(631) 421-1866

Irvington
Bella Flex Studio
adlerm@email.msn.com
(914) 591-5690
Nancy Adler, Instructor

Katonah
Equipoise at Barnspace
Carol Dodge Baker, Inst.
Teacher of T.
 113 Todd Road
Katonah, NY 10536
Instructors: Vandy Lipman,
Iris Salomon
(914) 232-3689 Fax: (914)
234-9289

Katonah
Iris Salomon, Instructor
Barnspace@mindspring.com
(914) 232-2034

Kingston
The Movement Center
Leah Chaback Feldman,,
Inst. Teacher. of T.
39 Broadway
Kingston, NY 12401
Instructors : Elise Bacon,
Beth Sullivan
(914) 331-0986

Lake Placid
Peak Edge Performance Inc.
Lake Placid, NY 12946
Karen Courtland Kelly,
Instructor
(518) 523-8706

Locust Valley
(Long Island)
Fitness Studio at Marathon
22 Forest Avenue
Locust Valley, NY 11560
Instructors: Doug Pollack,
Amy Wilson, Linda Figlia
(516) 671-8631

Locust Valley
Linda Figlia, Instructor
(718) 224-1695
Fra6301in@aol.com

Mt. Kisco
The Art of Control
Simona Cipriani, Instructor
37 West Main Street
Mt. Kisco, NY 10569
Instructors: Tiziana Trovati
Megan Bridge
(914) 242-0234

New Paltz
Elise Bacon, Instructor
12 North Chestnut Street
New Paltz, NY 12561
(914) 255-0559

Port Washington
Susan Brilliant, Instructor
(516) 883-8298

Port Washington
Total Body Dynamics
Patricia O'Donnell,
Instructor, Owner
(516) 944-0670

Rhinebeck
Deni Bank, Instructor
Astor Square Mall
Rhinebeck, NY 12572
88 Rt. 9N Suite 20
(845) 876-5114

Riverdale
Kerri Donegan, Instructor
(718) 548-1175

Rye
(Westchester County)
Amy Aronson Studio
560 Polly Park Road
Rye, New York 10580
(914) 921-0522
Amy Aronson, Instructor

Saratoga Springs
Lisa Hoffmaster, P.T
Instructor
376 Broadway, Suite 5
Saratoga Springs, NY 02866
(518) 677-2557

Scarsdale
Center for Movement
Owner/Instructor: Elle
Jardim, Donna Krystofiak
846 Scarsdale Avenue
Scarsdale, NY 10543
(914) 722-7646
Instructors: Michelle
Peperone, Marta Ferreria
Jean McCabe, Kathy Wolfe,
Tracy Fiore, Heather Synder

Sleepy Hollow
Saro Vanasup,
Owner/Instructor
(914) 524-9655
(Westchester County)

Southampton
Jeanette Davis, Instructor
395 County Road #39A
Southampton, NY 11968
(631) 204-0122

St. Albans
Miyuki Kato, Instructor
194-09 109th Avenue, #1F
St. Albans, NY 11412
Miyuki
mclaurine@cwix.com
(718) 217-9814

West Hampton
Mary McGuire Wein,
Instructor
(516) 325-3491

Woodbury
Tracy Greenfield, Instructor
Woodbury, NY
(516) 319-4915

Yonkers
Tracy Fiore, Instructor
DancerT@aol.com

NEW YORK CITY
(Inwood)
Rebecca Winters, Instructor
New York, NY 10034
(Nothern Tip of N.Y.C.)
(212) 340-4761

Jackson Heights
Renee Peters, Instructor
(718) 457-7980

(West Side)
Anne Walzel, Instructor
(713) 545-7061
The Pilates Studio
2121 Broadway, Suite 201
New York, NY 10023

(West Side)
Sean P. Gallagher PT, Dir.
(between 74th & 75th Str.)
(212) 875-0189
Fax: 769-2368
Instructors: Kelly Hogan,
Saro Vanasup, Brett Howard
Ton Voogt, Michael Fritzke,
Peter Fiasca, Sandra Zeuner
Sharon Henry, Junghee
Kallander, Molly Niles,
Brian Eshleman
Kerri Donegan, Nancy
Adler, Wendy Oliver,
Cristina Gallio

(West Side)
Cynthia Khoury, Instructor
2130 Broadway, #1002
New York, NY 10023
(212) 787-0746

(West Side)
Sharyl Curry, Instructor
(212) 316-3232

(West Side)
Mathilde M. Klein, P.T.,
Instructor
210 West 78th Street #3A
New York, NY 10023
(212) 595-3863

(West Side)
Reebok Sports Club
160 Columbus Avenue
New York, NY 10023
Instructors: Monique
Rhodriquez , Holly Cosner
(212) 501-3685
Sharon Korty

(West Side)
Alicia Principe, Instructor
210 West 101st Street
New York, NY 10025
(212) 662-6025

(West Side)
Suzanne Jordan, Instructor
55 West 111th St
New York, NY 10026
szanjord@usa.com
(212) 427-5238

(West Side)
Heather Snyder, Instructor
Hsnyder2@yahoo.com
(212) 396-9397

(Upper West Side)
Sandra Zeuner, Instructor
(212) 663-0688

(West Side)
Christina Richards,
Instructor
(212) 362-8939

(West Side)
Kim Reis, Instructor
Kikireis@aol.com
(212) 353-6813

(West Side)
Simone Cardoso, Instructor
(212) 582-9567

(West Side)
Monique Rhodriquez,
Instructor
(212) 222-4856

(West Side)
Junghee Kallander,
Instructor
Nabi0@aol.com
(212) 665-0575

(West Side)
Katrina Borgstrom,
Instructor
(917) 405-8659

(West Side)
Lori Oshansky, Instructor
138 West 74th Street, #A
New York, NY 10023
(212) 580-3746

(West Side)
Lara Serventi, Instructor
(212) 262-4721 VM: 626-
228-7601

(Midtown)
Drago's Gymnasium
50 West 57th Street, 6th
Floor
New York, NY 10019
(212) 757-0724
**Romana Kryzanowska,
Master Teacher**
Sari Pace, Master Teacher
Instructors: Lori Oshansky,
Jeanne Gross, Daria Pace,
Claude Assante, Jennifer
Holmes, Cynthia Shipley,
New York, NY 10111

(Midtown)
Wendy Stambler, Instructor
(212) 218-7333

(East Side)
**The Pilates Studio
& Pilates, Inc.**
890 Broadway, 6th FL
New York, NY 10003
Elyssa Rosenberg,
Associate Director
(212) 358-7676 Fax: 7678
(800) 474-5283 or
(888) 474-5283
Instructors: Stephanie
Beatty, Suzanne Jordan,
Brett Howard

(East Side)
Lynne Martens, Instructor
Waybox@aol.com
(917) 623-0245

(East Side)
**Premier Physical Therapy &
Wellness**
238 East 77th Street
New York, NY 10021
Joe Tatta, Instructor
(212) 249-5332

(East Side)
Makiko Oka, Instructor
East 60th Street
(212) 308-0786
MakikoOka@aol.net

(East Side)
JRW Physical Therapy
Roberta Wein, PT, Instruc.
60 East 56th Street, 5th Fl
New York, NY 10022
(212) 688-6089
Instructors: Yohanna Ragins,
Bernadette Ceravolo
Heather Simmons, Dyane
Harvey
RaWein1@aol.com

(East Side)
Geela Roland, Instructor
(212) 754-9071

(East Side)
Cristina Gregori, Instructor
cristi1009@aol.com
(212) 477-6288

(East Side)
Pamela Pardi, Instructor
ppardi5700@aol.com
(212) 420-5925

(East Side,UN)
Christy Ann Brown,
Instructor
(212) 973-0273

(West Village)
James Duus, Instructor
245 West 14th Street @ 8th
Ave.
(212) 229-7674

(Greenwich Village)
Diane Lam, Instructor
526 Hudson Street #2F
New York, NY 10014
Difijen@aol.com
(212) 627-8605

(Greenwich Village)
Village Body Mechanics
Clain Dipalma, Instructor
New York, NY 10011
(212) 229-9369

(NoHo)
Brooke Siler, Owner
33 Bleecker Street
@Mott Street, Suite 2C
New York, NY 10012
(212) 420-9111
Fax: (212) 475-4103
Instructors: Daniela Ubide,
Jennifer Ruggiero,
Karin Weidner, Amy Wilson,
Nikkie Eager
Ivanna Wei, Maria Hassabi,
Frances Craig,
Heather Snyder, Tracy
Fiore, Heather Simmons
Lisa Mathison

(SoHo)
Halle Markle, Instructor
594 Broadway (near
Houston Street) #904
New York, NY 10012
(212) 431-8377

(SoHo)
Frances Craig, Instructor
(212) 925-4629
Fcraig2@aol.com

(TriBeCa)
TriBeCa Bodyworks
Alycea Baylis,
Instructor/Owner
177 Duane St
New York, NY 10013
Instructors: Elizabeth
Knock, Gina Papalia
(212) 625-0777
Fax: (212) 625-0030
PilatesNYC@aol.com
Diane Lam, Hanne Koren,
Angeline Shaka,
Alison Thiem, Kathy
Buccellato, Tiziana Trovati
Gabrielle Gregory, Rosanna
Barberio, Rebecca Winters

NORTH CAROLINA
Asheville
Kathie Campbell, Instructor
(828) 285-9609
abeldon@aol.com

Boone
Marianne Adams, Instructor
665 Tarleton Circle
Boone, NC 28607
(828) 262-3028
Adamsm@appstate.edu

Chapel Hill
Celeste Neal Huntington,
Instructor
251 S. Elliot Road
Chapel Hill, NC 27514
(919) 929-1536

Huntersville
**Northeast Health
& Fitness Inst.**
Stephanie Weiner,
Instructor
1665 Birkdale Commons Pkwy
Huntersville, NC 28078
(704) 895-7048

Wilmington
The Studio
Ben Harris, Instructor
7210 Wrightsville Ave
Wilmington, NC 28403
(910) 509-1414 Fax: 0116

OHIO
Athens
The Body In Mind Studio
Instructors: Marina Walchli,
Leah Jean Rutkowski, Kris
Kumfer,
9 Factory Street
Athens, OH 45701
(740) 592-6090
Mwalchli:1@ohiou.edu

Athens
Leah Jean Rutkowski,
Instructor
11 Hocking St
Athens, OH 45701
(740) 589-6514
LR202595@oak.cats.ohiou.edu

Athens
Kris Kumfer, Instructor
Athens, OH 45701
(740) 597-6311

Centerville
Body Mind Flex
17 N. Main Street
Centerville, OH 45458
Cathy Stahura, Instructor
Ste.19A
(937) 439-9995

Cincinnati
Pam Medvecky, Instructor
Pamwmed@visto.com

OKLAHOMA
Norman
Laura Wren, Instructor
4017 Oxford Way
Norman, OK
(405) 321-6171

OREGON
Eugene
Susan Tate, Instructor
(541) 484-4011

Clackamas
Diane Caldwell, Instructor
dcaldwell@imagina.com
(503) 698-4613

Portland
Studio Adrienne, Inc.
Adrienne Silveria, Instructor
614 S.W. 11th Avenue
Portland, OR 97205
Roxane Murata, Teacher
Trainer
(503) 227-1470
Diane Caldwell, Instructor
ELN/ro22@earthlink.net

Portland
Wellspring Fitness Inc.
Anne Egan, Instructor
3424 NE 24th Avenue
Portland, OR 97212
(503) 249-0823
Anne_Egan@Juno.com

PENNSYLVANIA

Ambler
Peter Fiasca, Instructor
208 Brookwood Drive
Ambler, PA 19002
(215) 205-8004
Fax: 283-9063
pete-f@msn.com

Bryn Mawr
**The Pilates Studio
of Bryn Mawr**
899 Penn Street
Bryn Mawr, PA 19010
Megan Egan, Director, Inst.
(610) 581-0222
Fax: 610-581-0223

Doylestown
Physalchemy
22-28 S. Main Street, 2nd Fl
Doylestown, PA 18901
Zahra Nasser, Instructor
Zahra@voicenet.com
(215) 230-0787

Honesdale
Stone Gate Studio
Robin Dodson, Instructor
(570) 251-9408

Newtown
Caroline Nolan Probst,
Instructor
canopro@yahoo.com
Newtown, PA
(215) 598-8846 Fax: 8847

Philadelphia
**The Pilates Studio
@ the P.A. Ballet**
1101 South Broad Street
Philadelphia, PA 19147
June Hines, Instructor,
Megan Egan, Instructor
(215) 551-7000 ext. 1303
Fax: 7224

Philadelphia
Brie Neff, Instructor
brieadina@earthlink.com
(215) 545-3354

Philadelphia
Megan Bridge, Instructor
meganbridge@flashcom.net
(215) 925-0244

Pittsburgh
Dilla Mastrangelo & J.
Christopher Potts
820 Maryland Ave
Pittsburgh, PA 15232
Instructors
(412) 363-3426

Pittsburgh
Lynn Rescigno, Instructor
Pittsburgh, PA 15206
(412) 441-0774

Rydal
June Hines, Instructor
1132 Dixon Lane
Rydal, PA 19046
(215) 576-8261

State College
Terri Roberts, Instructor
terriroberts@hotmail.com
State College, PA 16803

Wilkes - Barre
Rose Ann Serpico,
Instructor
Rserp@prodigy.net
Wilkes-Barre, PA 18702
(570) 824-4391

Titusville
The Rankin Studio
Zane Rankin, Instructor
50A River Drive
Titusville, PA
(609) 730-9544

RHODE ISLAND

Barrington
Cassy DaSilva, Instructor
C1Angels@aol.com
Barrington, RI 02806
(401) 247-2700

East Greenwich
Body Mind Fitness, Inc.
Deborah Montaquila,
Instructor
5 Division Street East
East Greenwich, RI 02818
(401) 885-2102

Johnston
Balanced Fitness
Linda Chavaree, Instructor
1665 Hartford Avenue #36
Johnston, RI 02919
(401) 528-1166

Providence
Body By Design, Inc.
Catherine Cuzzone,
Instructor
126 Bayard Street
Providence, RI 02906
(401) 421-7408

Warwick
P. Turner Studio at R.G.E.
1775 Bald Hill Road
Warwick, RI 02886
Pamela Turner, Instructor
(401) 738-4401

SOUTH CAROLINA

Anderson
Edgar Tirado, Instructor
Camp Lou Ann
(864) 226-5439

Columbia
Ann Lore, Instructor
128 Woodshore Court
Columbia, SC 29223
(803) 788-7764
angelannsc@webtv.net

TENNESSEE

Franklin
Carrie Chrestman Leal,
Instructor
Franklin, TN
(615) 579-6688

Memphis
Bodies In Motion
Sway Hodges, Instructor
5111 Sanderlin Avenue
Memphis, TN 38117
(901) 452-4976

Nashville
Springs Studio
Julie Kraft, Instructor
2021 21st Avenue South,
Ste.100
Nashville, TN 37212
(old St.Bernards convent
bldg)
(615) 292-1930

Nashville
Bodies in Balance
1907-B Division Street
Nashville, TN 37203
Instructors: Sylvia
Gamonet, Grete Teague
2nd Floor
(615) 321-5100 Fax (5107)
Elizabeth McCoyd

Nashville
Grete Gryzwana Teague,
Instructor
epiphanydance@mind-
spring.com
(615) 321-5100

Nashville
Willow Studio
Bambi Watt, Instructor
5133 Harding Road
Nashville, TN 37205
(615) 354-1955

TEXAS

Austin
Body Springs Studio
Vicki Hickerson, Instructor
1912 West Anderson Lane
Austin, TX 78757
www.bodysprings.com
Suite 207
(512) 452-0115
vicki@bodysprings.com
Fax: (512) 453-8619

Austin
The Hills Fitness Center
Tracy Anderson, Instructor
4615 Beecaves Road
Austin, TX 78746
(512) 327-4881

Dallas
Body Proof Inc.
Read Gendler, Instructor
6706 Northaven Road
Dallas, TX 75230
(214) 369-7273 Fax: 7990

Galveston
Studio 424
Vicki Bolen, Instructor
424 22nd Street
Galveston, TX 77550
(409) 762-1399

UTAH

Orem
Physiques
1156 South State Street,
Ste. 206
Orem, UT 84097
James Urianza, Instructor
www.Jimurianza@aol.com
(801) 319-0383

Salt Lake City
Katie Howard, Instructor
2396 East Logan Way
Salt Lake City, UT 84108
(801) 582-4848

Body & Mind Studio
Salt Lake City
Claudia Flores, Instructor
3300 South 1063 East,
Suite 201
Salt Lake City, UT 84106
Sondra Fair, Instructor
(801) 486-2660

VIRGINIA

Arlington
Body Logic
3017 B Clarendon Blvd.
Arlington, VA 22201
Karen Garcia, Instructor
Diane Popper,
Simi Nary Instructors
Studiobodylogic@eartlink.net
(703) 527-9626

Herndon
Classical Ballet Academy
Mat class only
Chris Abbott, Instructor
320 Victory Drive
Herndon, VA 20170
(703) 471-0750

Norfolk
Power House
134 W. Olney Road
Norfolk, VA 23510
Camilo Rodriguez & Todd
Rosenlieb, Instructors
(757) 622-4822

Reston
Pure Joe Studios
2254-M Hunters Woods
Village Center
Reston, VA 20191
Michael Rooks, Instructor
Andrea Chastant, Instructor
(703) 860-6766

Richmond
4S Fitness, Inc.
2927A West Cary Street
Richmond, VA 23221
Jerry Weiss, Instructor
jweissguy@altavista.com
(804) 355-5010

Virginia Beach
Studio P.
4020 Bonney Road, Ste. 104
Virginia Beach, VA 23452
Leslie Vise-Clark, Instructor
Reid Strasma, Instructor
(757) 306-7007 Fax 7009

Virginia Beach
AXIOM
Chambord Commons
Virginia Beach, VA 23454
Elyse Tapper Cardon,
Instructor
332 N. Great Neck Road,
Suite 105
(757) 486-8665 FAX: 8663
davelyse@aol.com

WASHINGTON, D.C.
Excel Movement Studio
3407 8th Street NE
2nd Floor
Washington, D.C. 20017
(202) 269-3020
Instructors: Lesa McLaughlin
Kerry Devivo,
Christine Abbott
Dianne Signiski Garrett,
Jill Kuhlman

Fitness For Life
Instructor: Brigitte Ziebell
1417 27th ST NW
Washington, D.C. 20007
(202) 338-6765

WASHINGTON STATE
Everett
**Intrinsic Energy
Studio**Bernadette Wilson,
Instructor
3426 Broadway, Ste. 301A
Everett, WA 98201
(425) 252-8240

Kirkland
Atasha Avery, Instructor
429 8th Ave
Kirkland, WA 98033
Atasha_a@hotmail.com
(206) 822-2448

Seattle
The Pilates Studio Seattle
& Capitol Hill Physical
Therapy
413 Fairview Ave. North
Seattle, WA 98109
(206) 405-3560 Fax: (3938)
Lauren Stephen,
Director-Instructor
Lori Coleman- Brown, PT,
Director-Instructor
Dorothee Vandewalle,
Teacher
Instructors: Bernadette
Wilson, Anje Marshall, Joe
Nicoli, Marywilde Nelson,
Sachiko Glass PT, ChaCha
Guerrero, Danielle Stanley,
Teresa Shupe, Laurel
Levasheff

Seattle
Robert Leonard Spa
Instructors: Christl Siris,
Rick Morris, Anje Marshall
2033 6th Avenue
Seattle, WA 98121
(206) 441-9900
www.Robertleonard.com

Seattle
Dorothee Vandewalle,
Teacher of Teacher, Inst.
Seattle, WA 98105
(206) 526-0155

Seattle
Jennifer Saltzman,
Instructor
915 E. Pine Street #408
Seattle, WA 98112
(206) 726-1903

Shoreline
Peggy Z. Protz, Instructor
102 N. 171st Street
Shoreline, WA 98133
pez009@sttl.uswest.net
(206)533-0820

WISCONSIN
Milwaukee
Body Mechanics Studio
807 N. Jefferson
Milwaukee, WI 53202
Jennifer Goldbeck,
Instructor
(414) 224-8219

WYOMING
Jackson
Sally Lynne Baker,
Instructor
P.O.B 10609
Jackson, WY 83002
(307) 734-8940
DLCrawf@aol.com

Teton Village
Interhealth Studio
Sally Baker, Instructor
P.O.B 10609
Jackson, WY 83002
(307) 734-8940
Fax: (307) 733-0391

International Instructors Certified by The Pilates Studio

AUSTRALIA
Surry Hills
The New York Pilates
Studio ® of Australia
Director, Inst. Cynthia
Lochard.
Suite 12, Level 4/46-56
Tel / Fax: 011 612 9698-4689
Instructors: Roula
Kantarzoglou
Holt Street,
Surry Hills, 2010 Australia
Edwina Ward
www.pilatesm.com

Rozelle
**Powerhouse Personal
Training**
Instructors: Gina Richter &
Chris Lavelle
PO Box 179
Rozelle, NSW 2137
Tel: 011 612 9818 6234
powerhouse@hotkey.net.au
Fax: 011 612 98186235

Sydney
Paulina Quinteros,
Instructor
4/1 St Neot Ave
Tel: 011-612-9357 7448
Potts Point, Sydney 2011
Pquinteros@hotmail.com

Sydney
Lisa Mathison, Instructor
Lisamath@hotmail.com

Sydney
Maria Persenitis, Instructor
Tel: 011-411-870-468

AUSTRIA
Gabriella Cimino, Instructor
Performing Arts Studios
Vienna
Tel/Fax: 011431 523 5656
Zieglergasse 7, 1070 Vienna
Austria

BRAZIL
Sao Paulo
The Pilates Studio Brazil
Rua Januario Matroni,
194 Vila das Palmerias
Guarulhos, Sao Paulo, Brazil
CEP 07024-070
Tel/Fax: 011-551-164240244
Inelia Ester G. Garcia
Kolyniak, Director/ Inst.
Adriana Trotti Banci,
Instructor
ineliagarcia@hotmail.com

Sao Paulo
The Pilates Studio Brazil
R. Oscar Freire, 2066
Cerqueira Cesar
Sao Paulo, Brazil CEP
05409-011
Tel: 011 551 1 3061 0647
Inelia Ester G. Garcia
Kolyniak, Director/ Inst.
Instructors: Alfonso
Fernando Carrillo,
Roberta Alves Cardona

Sao Paulo
Bergson Queiroz, Instructor
Rua Herculano de Freitas
237-Ap 187
Sao Paulo, SP Brazil
01308-020
Tel: 011- 55-11-234-5106
Certified for USA

Sao Paulo
Marta Ferreira, Instructor
Tel: 011 5514 43333947
E-mail: jamela@dori.com.br
Certified for USA

Porto Alegre
Studio Balance
Alessandra Tegoni,
Instructor
Av. Encantado, 410
Porto Alegre-RS 90470-420
Tel: 011-555-1330-6346

BERMUDA
Hamilton
Jackie Jinks, Instructor
Suite 1002 48 Para La Ville
Road Tel: (441) 293-0127
Jinskytwo@ibl.bm

Hamilton
Contrology! Bermuda Ltd.
Suite 1147
48 Parla-Ville Road
Hamilton, Bermuda HM11
Sophia Cannonier,
Instructor
Tel: 441-291-5895
Fax: 441-236-7998

CANADA
Calgary
Body Dynamics
Lynne Smith, Instructor
924 17th Avenue SW
Tel: 403-244-4448
Calgary, Alberta Canada
T2T0A2

Montreal
Deja Griffith, Instructor
#414 3025 Sherbrook
Street West
Tel: 514-989-8299
Montreal, Quebec H3Z-1A1
Montreal
Therese Desrosiers,
Instructor
Schehera_zade@hotmail.com

Ontario
Michaela Sirbu, Instructor
London, Ontario
Tel: 519-457-1371
mcs@lon.ionline.net

CHILE
Santiago |
Marcela Ortiz De Zarate
Broughton, Instr.
El Buen Camino 9680 8-B
Penalolen, Santiago Chile
Tel / Fax: 011 562 292 7485
Maoritz2000@hotmail.com

CHINA
Hong Kong
Louise Crawley, Instructor
Discovery Bay, Hong Kong
Tel: 011-852-2987-0976
crawleylouise@hotmail.com

ENGLAND
Cornwall
(4 hours from London)
Gayla Zukevich Stulce,
Instructor
6 Meadow Rise
St. Columbus Major
Cornwall, UK TR9 6BL
Tel: 011 441 637881972
meadowrise@aol.com

205

London
Daphne Pena Higgs,
Instructor
E Mail:
daphnepena@hotmail.com

FRANCE
Marseille
Monica Germani, Instructor
23 Rue de la Guadelupe
13006 Marseille France
Tel: 011 91 71 0303

Paris
Phillipe Taupin, Instructor
Le Centre Du Marais
39 Rue Du Temple
75004 Paris France
Tel: 011-331-427-29174
Fax: 011-331-427-29187

GERMANY
Berlin
Galina Rohleder, Instructor
Schluterstrasse 13
10625 Berlin Germany
Tel / Fax: 011 49 30 823 1124

Berlin
Eduardo Laranjeira,
Instructor
Stargarder Str. 12
Tel: 011 49 30 444 5276
10437 Berlin Germany
elaranjeir@aol.com

Frankfurt
Leigh Matthews, Instructor
Mayra Rodriguez de
Matthews, Instructor
Hans-Thoma-Strasse 7 (H.h)
60596 Frankfurt
Tel/Fax: 011 49 69 603 2156

Munich
Karin Weidner-Mubanda,
Instructor
Tel: 011 49 89 957 6841

Stuttgart
Davorka Kulenovic,
Instructor
Sickstr. 32 / 70190,
Stuttgart Germany
Tel: 011 497 11 9239026

GREECE
Athens
Eugenia Papadopolou,
Instructor
Corpus Ray,
4 Doxapatri Street
114 71 Athens- Greece
Tel: 011 301 361 7290

Cyprus
Emily Papaloizou, Instructor
Tel: 011-357-534 2582

ICELAND
Reykjavik
**National School of Ballet
in Iceland**
Lisa S.T. Johannsson,
Instructor
Engjateig 1
Reykjavik 105, Iceland
Fax: 011-354-557-2948
Tel: 011 354-553-0660

ITALY
Verona
Contrology Studio Italia
Karin Cid, Director, Instruc.
Via San Pietro Incamario, 4
37121 Verona, Italy
Tel: 011 39 0329 2244764
Fax: 011 39 0442 607000
www.contrology.it
pilates@contrology.it

JAPAN
Tokyo
Yumi Takada, Instructor
University of the Sacred
Heart
Hiroo 4 Chome 3-1
Shibuya-Ku, Tokyo, Japan
Tel: 011 813 548 53884

Tokyo
Makiko Oka, Instructor
2-59-6 Ikebukuro
Toshima-Ku, Tokyo
Japan 171
Tel: 011 813 984-6546

LATVIA
Rtga
Aija Peagle, Instructor
Studija Sports Pluss
Blaumanu iela 5A
Rtga, Latvia

NETHERLANDS
The Hague
(BeNeLux)
The New York Pilates
Studio of the Netherlands
Owner /Instructor:
Marjorie Oron
Inst. Jane Poerwoatmodjo
Keizerstraat 32
2584 BJ The Hague,
Netherlands
Tel: 011 31 703 508 684
Fax: 011 31 703 228285
e-mail: Marjorie@pilates.nl

Rosmalen
Marjon Van Grunsven,
Instructor
JanHeymanslaan 139
5246 BK Rosmalen
Tel: 011 317 3641 8956
Voicemail (212) 726-8436

NORWAY
Oslo
Lene Danielsen, Instructor
lenedani@hotmail.com
Tel: 011 47-23220080

PHILIPPINES
Manila
Cecile Sicangco Ibarrola,
Instructor
227 Reposo Street
Bel Air II, Makati
Manila, Philippines 1209
Tel: 011 632 895 4465

PORTUGAL
Lisbon
Maria dos Anjos Machado
Rua.de Angola, blc-6, 3-A
Encosta Da Carreira
2750 Cas Cais, Portugal
Tel: 011-351-14865652

SOUTH AFRICA
Houghton
Natasha Madel, Instructor
Tel: 011 2711 4830768

SOUTH AMERICA
Santiago, Chile
Fransisca Molina, Instructor
Nueva Costanera 4076
Tel/ Fax: 011 562 228 7133
Santiago, Chile

SPAIN
Madrid
Estudio Lara
Lara Fermin, Instructor
C/ Magallanes 28, 1 A
28015 Madrid Spain
Tel/Fax: 011 349 159 43863

SWITZERLAND
Sophie Morabia, Instructor
Tel: 011 33 450 388195

The Pilates® Method

Official Apparatus of the Pilates Studio

All prices are approximate and subject to change. To order or to get more information: Call Toll-Free: 1-888-278-7227 or 1-845-357-1383.
Or visit the website at: www.pilates-studio.com

THE MAT

Basic Floor Mat (20" x 54" x .5") plus 11-minute video $39.99 + $7.50 S&H

Basic Mat Video without Mat 11 minutes $24.99 + $5.75 S&H

Intermediate Mat Video 30 minutes $29.99 + $5.75 S&H

Advanced Mat Video 50 minutes $29.99 + $5.75 S&H

MAGIC CIRCLE

Magic Circle & 15 minute video $29.99 + $6.50 S&H

PILATES PERFORMER™

Dimensions: (Open) 7'2" long; 20" wide; 17" high

Dimensions: (Closed) 45" long; 20" wide; 8" high without foot rollers

Basic Video and workout chart included.
    BASIC MODEL $369.00 + $44.00 S&H
    DELUXE CHERRY WOOD MODEL $449.00 + $50.00 S&H

Intermediate Performer Video 25 minutes $29.99 + $5.75 S&H

Advanced Performer Video 45 minutes $29.99 + $5.75 S&H

Box, Pole & Video for the Performer: $99.99 + $20.00 S&H

LARGE & SMALL BARRELS

Not yet available.

Price not yet set. Please call to inquire.

SPRINGS & HOOK ATTACHMENTS

Not yet available.

Price not yet set. Please call to inquire.

THE CHAIR

Not yet available.

Price not yet set. Please call to inquire.

PILATESWEAR

Workout Clothing for Men and Women

See the website at www.pilates-studio.com or call.

General Index

The Pilates® Method